Throat Cancer Diary

This Has to Become Useful

WRITTEN BY

RYAN BUETER

Throat Cancer Diary

This book reflects the author's present recollections of experiences over time. Some names and identifying details may have been changed. Dialogue has been recreated from memory.

USA Publishing Hub

New York

First Edition

For my Mother the English teacher

For my Father the singer

For my keepers, Rick, Mark, and Sean

For Jenn

For Joan

For The Patches

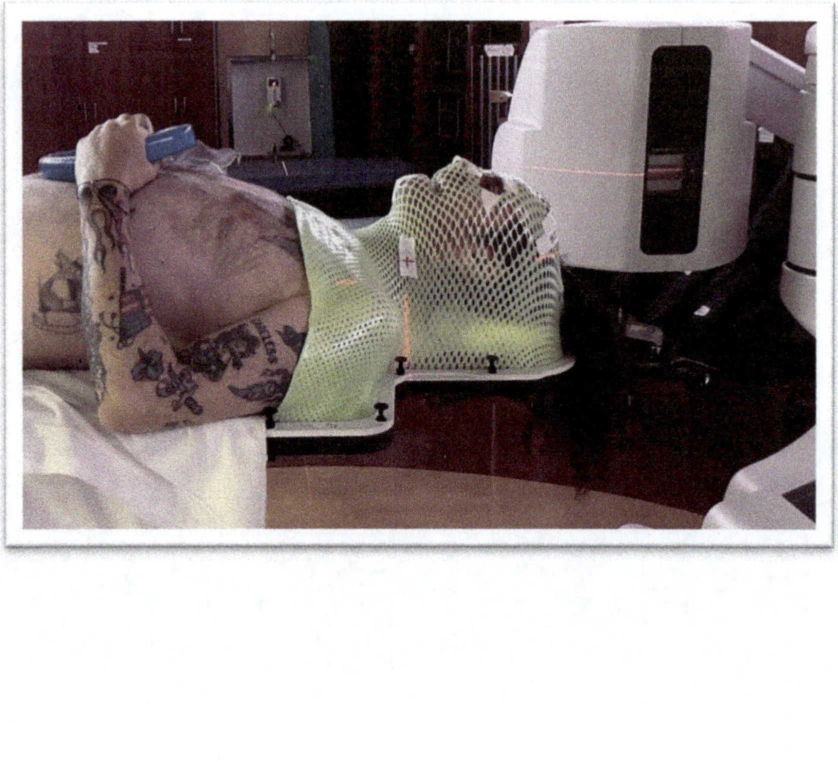

Author's Note

I've always felt biographies were a bit self-indulgent. To think any of our lives are so special that we feel someone should hear our story makes my stomach turn. When I got sober, so many people told me I should write a book, but I didn't feel sobriety was something I should get a pat on the back for. When I got throat cancer, and being a singer, even before treatment began, I felt a calling to tell my story in hopes someone could be helped by it.

Contents

CHAPTER ONE

The Email

MARCH 28, 2025 — 3:30 P.M.

"Give me love, give me hope, give me strength, give me someone to live for."

SONG: STRENGTH
BAND: THE ALARM

Squamous cell carcinoma positive for p16.

That was the first line of the email. Not "We're sorry." Not "Please call your doctor." Not even a human voice explaining what I was about to read. Just those words sitting in a pathology report that arrived in my inbox at 3:30 p.m. on Friday, March 28, 2025. I wasn't expecting the results until Monday.

Ten days earlier, on March 19, a surgeon had removed a tumor from the right side of my neck. It had coiled around my jugular vein and pushed up near the base of my skull. At the time, nobody seemed overly concerned. The ENT told me he wasn't particularly worried. The tumor would be sent to pathology, and the following Monday he would call me to discuss the findings. There was no need for me to come back in. There was no urgency in his tone and nothing in that conversation that prepared me for what eventually showed up in my email.

I had a post-op visit on March 24. They removed the drainage tube from my neck and checked the incision. I had thirty stitches pulling every time I swallowed. I was sore, but stable. I continued managing performances for my business, The Killer Dueling Pianos, remotely. My teams were performing while I recovered. I wasn't ready to get back onstage yet, and I had a scar that looked like it came from a knife fight, but there was still a business to run.

Nothing on the surface seemed particularly alarming, but underneath all of it, I knew something wasn't right. Hell, even my cat Smokey knew, but we'll get to that later.

The first sign had come months earlier. Back in October 2024, I started feeling something strange around my right tonsil. It felt like a corn kernel was stuck back there. It was subtle, annoying, and easy for someone else to dismiss. And doctors did dismiss it. I was told it was COVID. Then strep. Then nothing.

But I knew.

There is a difference between anxiety and instinct. I know anxiety. Anxiety can be loud as hell. It can convince you of things that aren't happening and keep you trapped in your own head. This felt different. For weeks and weeks, I had the feeling that something was wrong. I couldn't prove it. I didn't have the medical language to explain it. I only knew my own body, and I knew the sensation around my right tonsil wasn't normal.

Then, in January, the tumor popped out in my neck.

By then, the people closest to me knew what had been happening. My parents knew. My brothers Rick, Mark, and Sean knew. My friend Dr. Chris Wray knew and had been following the situation closely. Chris and I had been talking quite a bit since the tumor appeared. He knew about the surgery and wanted updates. We were all waiting for the pathology results. We thought we would get them Monday.

Instead, the email arrived Friday afternoon.

I opened the attachment and read the report again. **Squamous cell carcinoma positive for p16.** I wasn't completely familiar with the medical terminology, but I knew enough to understand the words that mattered. Carcinoma. Cancer. Positive. I read it again, and then I read it again.

I had not been prepared for this. The ENT had not seemed worried. I had been told I would get a phone call on Monday. Now I was sitting at home with thirty stitches in my neck, looking at a pathology report that appeared to be telling me I had cancer. There was no explanation, no context, and no doctor attached to it. Just the report.

I called the hospital. At that point, I needed someone to tell me whether I was understanding what I had just read. I wanted clarification. I wanted a doctor to explain what "positive for p16" meant and what I was supposed to do next. Someone answered, but not someone who could do anything. My doctor was gone for the day.

I asked if I could speak to the ENT on call. The answer was no. I tried to get someone else to talk to me, anyone who could look at the pathology report and tell me what it meant. Nobody would. I was told I would have to wait until Monday, when my doctor came back.

Wait until Monday?

That was when I became angry as hell. You just sent me a pathology report that says I have cancer. You sent it to me without warning at 3:30 on a Friday afternoon. I wasn't expecting the results until Monday. I am ten days out of surgery with thirty stitches in my neck, and I am sitting in my house trying to figure out whether I have cancer. I call the hospital that sent me the report, and nobody will talk to me. Now I'm supposed to wait until Monday?

How do they even do this to people and keep a good conscience?

I could not get past that. I wasn't panicking about dying. I was enraged by the way the diagnosis had been delivered and by the fact that the hospital had left me hanging after delivering it. If you're going to send someone a cancer diagnosis in an email, there has to be a human being available afterward. There has to be someone who understands that the pathology report they just released belongs to an actual person—a person with emotions, a person with a family, a person who is going to read the word *carcinoma* and immediately have questions.

Instead, I got an email, and then I got, "Wait until Monday."

Being diagnosed with something life-altering through an automated system is dehumanizing. There was no voice. No eye contact. No pause to let the information land. Nobody asking whether I understood what I was reading. At that moment, I didn't feel like a patient. I felt like a number.

That feeling was made worse by what had happened when I arrived at the hospital for surgery. I had been required to pay my full deductible up front—everything my insurance had not covered. The man and woman next to me were government-insured. They paid nothing. I paid to have a tumor removed from my neck. Ten days later, I found out I had cancer through an email. Then, when I called the hospital that sent the diagnosis, nobody would speak to me about it.

I was furious.

Throughout that afternoon and evening, I was communicating with my family. My parents were part of those conversations. So were my brothers, Rick, Mark, and Sean. They had been following what was happening with me. They knew about the strange feeling near my right tonsil. They knew about the tumor in my neck. They knew I had gone through surgery and that we were waiting for pathology. Now I was telling them the results had arrived early.

Cancer.

My family and I were trying to understand what the report meant and what was going to happen next. I wasn't quietly sitting alone with this information and keeping it from everyone. We were communicating throughout the day. I wasn't hysterical. I was angry. I was angry that I had been blindsided on a Friday afternoon. I was angry that the hospital had sent something this serious without warning. I was angry that, after receiving it, I couldn't get anyone there to talk to me.

And I still needed to know for certain whether the report meant what I thought it meant.

That's where Chris came in.

Chris Wray wasn't someone I suddenly called out of the blue because I happened to know a doctor. He had been following my situation closely since the tumor popped out in January. We had already spent quite a bit of time on the phone. He knew I was having surgery. He knew we were waiting for the pathology results. He wanted me to keep him updated.

Chris and I had known each other since I was fourteen years old. We became friends during my freshman year of high school in Dublin, Ohio. He was two years older than me. Chris played guitar. I played bass and sang lead. Along with our friend Dru Betts on drums, we formed a band called The Myst.

We practiced every chance we got—summers, weekends, garages. When I was sixteen, we recorded a two-song 45. I always looked up to Chris and Dru. They both seemed so much more confident than I was. I wanted to be like them. When you spend that much time chasing music with someone, especially when you're young, something forms. It isn't just a casual friendship. There is a brotherhood that stays with you.

Over the decades, our lives went in different directions. I became a professional musician. So did Dru. Chris became an anesthesiologist at UCLA. But we stayed in touch. We went to concerts together, especially to see our favorite band, Rush. Who would have guessed that forty years after high school I would need Chris not only as my friend, but also as a doctor?

I took photos of the pathology report and texted them to him. Chris wasn't surprised that I was calling him about my medical situation. He already knew what I had been going through. What surprised him was the email. He couldn't believe I had received a diagnosis like this on a Friday afternoon and then been told nobody at the hospital would discuss it with me until Monday.

"I'm going to call an ENT I know," he told me. "I'll call you right back."

I waited. When Chris called me back, his tone had changed. He sounded sad.

"I'm really sorry," he said. "I hate to say it, but this says you have cancer."

There it was. Not in an email. In a human voice.

As strange as it sounds, hearing Chris say the words was easier than reading them on a screen. Chris knew me. He knew what had been happening since January. He knew about the surgery and the pathology report. He understood the weight of what he was telling me. At least there was a person on the other end of the phone.

I didn't immediately think about death. My first thought was, *What am I going to do about my business?*

I had employees. Contracts. Shows booked months in advance. Payroll. Rent. Insurance. People depended on me. I didn't know anything about this type of cancer. I didn't know what treatment would look like. I didn't know the timeline. I didn't know how long I might be unable to perform. I didn't know the survival rates. I didn't know what was coming.

But I knew one thing: life doesn't stop just because you're sick.

My employees still had to be paid. The shows were still booked. The contracts still existed. My business wasn't going to stop running because the word *cancer* had appeared in my inbox.

Then another thought came back to me. During the darkest days of the pandemic in 2020, my industry collapsed and my girlfriend of five years left. I went into an emotional downward spiral. The darkest place I had ever been. During that period, I had a strange thought that I couldn't shake: if I didn't pull myself out of this, I was going to get cancer.

It wasn't logical. It wasn't medical. It was a premonition. I can't explain why I thought it. It was almost as if one day, I felt a change in my soul.

Now, five years later, here it was.

Cancer.

And it had arrived in an email.

The following Monday, I went to the ENT in person. I brought my business partner Donny and my friend Kim. We talked about treatment possibilities, scans, radiation, and options. But Chris was already moving.

Within a few days, he got me an appointment at UCLA Health. My case would be reviewed by the head of ENT there. Fresno was weeks, maybe months, behind on consultations. UCLA could see me within ten days.

The contrast was staggering. I had just spent an entire weekend knowing I had cancer because of an email and being unable to get anyone at the hospital to explain the diagnosis to me. Now I was being connected with people at UCLA who understood that speed mattered.

During those early days, I made one thing very clear to everyone around me. I was not interested in fighting insurance companies.

I had seen friends spend the last year of their lives tangled in red tape instead of living their final days. Phone calls. Arguments. Stress. They were already sick, and on top of being sick, they were fighting over coverage. They were angry, exhausted, and depressed.

I wasn't doing that.

I told my family and friends that if they wanted me alive, they needed to understand something: I was not wasting whatever time I had left arguing with someone on the phone at an insurance company. I meant it. I was at peace with God. If this was the path, so be it. What I was not at peace with was the idea that bureaucracy could steal whatever time remained.

But once UCLA stepped in, something remarkable happened. I never had to call the insurance company. Not once.

And something began to change inside me. The diagnosis itself didn't feel like a death sentence. It started to feel like a responsibility. Within two weeks, I had a realization.

This had to become useful.

In 2021, I participated in a Man of the Year campaign for the Leukemia & Lymphoma Society. Our fundraising team was called Ryan's Rockstars. At the beginning of the campaign, I told Donny we weren't finished with that name. I believed it meant something bigger. At the time, I didn't know what.

Now I was beginning to understand.

Cancer had entered my life. I could treat it entirely as a personal struggle. I could focus on myself, get through treatment, survive if I was fortunate enough to survive, and try to return to the life I had before.

Or I could turn it outward.

There are people walking around right now with symptoms they are ignoring because the symptoms don't seem serious enough. There are artists and musicians who push through pain because that's what we do. The show has to go on. There are patients who are afraid of their doctors or too intimidated to ask questions. There are people who don't know how to ask for help.

And there will be other people who open an email and read something that changes everything.

I needed my experience to mean something to them. Survival alone wasn't enough. I needed to be of service.

At 3:30 p.m. on Friday, March 28, 2025, I became a cancer patient. I didn't know what treatment was going to do to me. I didn't know what it would do to my voice. I didn't know what would happen to my business. I didn't know if I would live or die.

But somewhere in everything that followed that email, I understood that I had another responsibility. I had to tell the truth about what happened. I had to make it useful.

This story, whether I live or die, will not be self-indulgent.

It will be useful.

CHAPTER TWO

The Boy with the Insecurities

"We are, we are, we are but your children
Finding our way around indecision
We are, we are, we are rather helpless
Take us forever, a whisper to a scream"

SONG: BIRDS FLY (WHISPER TO A SCREAM)
BAND: THE ICICLE WORKS

I was raised in Dublin, Ohio, which, from the outside, seems like a stable place to grow up. My parents moved us there when I was seven years old. The neighborhood was still under construction then, with new streets being laid and new houses going up around us. It was the kind of place that gave you a sense of security.

My parents had not come from much, and neither of them had grown up with that same sense of security. My mother lost her father when she was twelve years old. Two years later, she watched her own mother suffer a debilitating stroke. My father also lost his father in his early 20s. They both learned early what it meant to have stability taken away from you.

Whatever security they wanted in life, they had to build themselves. They did it little by little, through discipline, sacrifice, and belief. By the time I was born, my parents had established themselves and created a home filled with stability, order, and affection. I knew my family loved me. I never questioned that.

But I always had an emptiness inside.

There were four of us boys, and I was the youngest. My oldest brother was almost a decade older than me, and the others weren't far behind him. We were close, but because of the age difference, we weren't always living the same life at the same time. My brothers were already developing their own interests and moving through the world with a kind of independence I hadn't reached yet.

I often felt like I was trying to catch up to something that had already passed me. Even inside my own family, where I knew I belonged and knew I was loved, there was still this feeling that I didn't completely fit. It wasn't something my parents or brothers had done to me. I just had this emptiness inside, and at that age, I had no idea what to call it.

I carried that feeling into school.

I remember walking into a new classroom when I was about eight years old and immediately feeling like I didn't belong. Nothing specific happened. Nobody said anything cruel to me. There was no incident that left me visibly shaken or some big traumatic moment I can point to and say, *That's where it started.*

I just felt it.

The other kids seemed to understand something I didn't. They knew how to socialize, how to find their place, and how to exist without questioning everything they did. At least, that's how it looked to me. I didn't have that same sense of comfort.

That feeling of being out of place didn't go away. It settled into me and became part of how I saw myself. I played sports, but I was never good enough to stand out. I was usually one of the last kids picked. It wasn't because people disliked me. There was just always someone else who seemed like a better choice.

I had friends. Real friends. But even with them, I kept a quiet distance that I didn't completely understand.

I could be laughing in a group of people and still feel disconnected. It's difficult to explain unless you've experienced it. I was physically there. I could participate in the conversation and have a good time, but part of me always seemed to be somewhere else, watching everything instead of completely living in it.

When you feel that way long enough, you start measuring yourself constantly. I looked for signs that confirmed what I already suspected about myself: that I wasn't quite enough, wasn't quite right, or wasn't where I was supposed to be. As a child, I didn't have the words or awareness to challenge those thoughts. I didn't know anything about insecurity or why my mind worked the way it did.

I just absorbed it.

For me, music was the first place where that feeling disappeared.

It started simply. When I was seven years old, my oldest brother Rick gave me a pair of drumsticks. There wasn't some big moment attached to it. Nobody handed me those drumsticks and announced that music was going to become my life. They were just a pair of drumsticks.

But something connected.

My parents noticed my interest and supported it in ways I didn't fully appreciate at the time. They drove me to drum lessons every week, even when it was inconvenient. They consistently showed up for me, but they didn't immediately go out and buy me a full drum set.

I had to earn that.

For the first year, I practiced on a practice pad. After a year, I got a single snare drum. Then, after two years of showing my parents I was serious, I finally got a full drum set.

I was serious. I just didn't know how to explain how serious I was.

After school, I would go straight to the drums. It wasn't about discipline or forcing myself to practice. Nobody had to tell me to sit down and play. I wanted to be there because it was one of the only places where my mind felt at ease.

All the confusion, insecurity, and self-doubt I carried around during the day would quiet down when I played. I wasn't wondering whether people liked me. I wasn't thinking about being picked last or trying to understand why everyone else seemed more comfortable than I was.

I was playing drums.

Music wasn't just an activity for me.

It was relief.

Music had always been part of my environment. My father had been a professional singer when he was younger and had performed on Ed Sullivan's *Toast of the Town* before I was born. My mother was trained in piano. Our house was always filled with music, so there was always a sense that music meant something in our family.

Over time, it became personal for me. It wasn't just something happening around me anymore.

It was something I needed.

Around the age of ten, that connection became even stronger. I started going through my brothers' old records and listening to anything I could find. Around that same time, John Lennon was murdered, and I was introduced to the Beatles.

I was ten years old. I didn't fully understand the cultural impact of the Beatles or everything John Lennon's death meant to people who had grown up with his music. I didn't know enough about music history to analyze any of it.

I just felt something when I listened.

There was a sense of completeness to the music. Something about it felt right to me, even though I couldn't explain why. The songs weren't just good.

They felt honest.

My drum teacher, Steve Dodge, started teaching me Beatles songs, and the first one I learned was "She Loves You." That stayed with me. There was something different about learning how to play a song instead of just listening to one. I wasn't only hearing music coming through a speaker anymore.

I was learning how to make it.

For a kid who spent so much time feeling like he didn't quite fit anywhere, that mattered. Learning a song felt like becoming something more. Something bigger than the insecure version of myself I carried around every day.

It gave me a sense of identity.

Music was no longer just something I listened to.

It became something I lived in.

As I got older, I started writing poetry and lyrics. I wrote anything that allowed me to express the things I didn't know how to say through actions or conversation. I knew I had thoughts and emotions that needed somewhere to go, and writing gave me that space.

I was also becoming more aware of how sensitive I was.

It didn't take much to affect me. A small argument could stay with me much longer than it probably should have. A harsh comment could get stuck in my head. Even a misunderstanding could become something I replayed and analyzed over and over until I had made it much bigger in my mind.

I held on to things.

Then came heartbreak.

Heartbreak is a normal part of growing up. Almost everybody goes through it. But when it happens to you for the first time, knowing that other people have survived it doesn't make it hurt any less.

I didn't know how to process that kind of pain. I didn't know how to let it go. It felt like something had been taken from me and left another empty space where something important had been.

I didn't want to disappear.

I just didn't know how to live with that kind of pain.

So I turned even more to music.

By high school, I was fully invested. I formed the band with Chris Wray on guitar, Dru Betts on drums, and me on bass guitar and lead vocals. We called ourselves The Myst. We practiced for hours and took every opportunity we could to play.

Of course we had stars in our eyes. We were young musicians. But it wasn't only about becoming famous.

We were chasing a feeling.

Nothing mattered more to me than performing. The moments I spent onstage were powerful because I wasn't insecure there. I didn't question myself. I didn't compare myself to anyone else or wonder whether I was good enough to be included.

I simply existed in the music.

Onstage, I felt like I belonged completely.

Offstage, nothing had really changed.

I still didn't know who I was. I still wanted to be liked. I avoided asking for help because I didn't want to be seen as a burden or an imposition. Somewhere along the way, I had developed a habit of walking on eggshells.

I adjusted myself to other people. I tried to keep things smooth. I avoided conflict whenever I could because I didn't want rejection. I didn't understand at the time how much that way of living could affect everything—your relationships, your sense of yourself, and eventually the way you see your future.

I wasn't aware of any of that then.

I was just searching for something to fill the empty space.

Music helped.

But it didn't solve everything.

By my sophomore year of high school, one thing had become clear to me. I wasn't going to follow a conventional path.

School felt like something I had to endure rather than something that was helping me grow. I struggled to focus on subjects that required constant reading or long periods of attention. It wasn't laziness. I could work hard when something mattered to me. The problem was that I felt completely disconnected from most of what I was being asked to do in school.

Music was different.

I could focus on music without effort. I could practice for hours without getting tired of it. Nobody had to stand over me and make sure I was doing the work.

Give me an instrument, and I was there.

School didn't work that way for me.

So I made a decision. I wasn't going to take the traditional path. I wanted to prove that I was serious about something else.

My parents didn't discourage me, but they also weren't going to accept it without question. They had built their lives through discipline and sacrifice. If I was telling them I wanted a different life, they wanted to see commitment.

So I showed them.

I took summer school classes so I could free up time during the regular school year. That gave me more room to focus on music and the band. I practiced constantly, not because I had to, but because music was still the one thing that felt completely right to me.

I started playing more shows and performing wherever I could. It wasn't glamorous. I wasn't suddenly famous. But I was moving forward.

It felt like progress.

At some point, I came across a brochure for a music school in Hollywood called Musicians Institute. The school focused entirely on music. Guitar. Bass. Drums. Vocals. Playing, studying, and creating in an environment built around the thing I cared about most.

There was no unnecessary coursework standing between me and what I wanted to learn.

The idea stayed with me.

Hollywood.

A school for musicians.

For the first time, the life I imagined didn't feel completely impossible. There was an actual place I could go. A place built around music and filled with people who wanted the same basic thing I did.

By my senior year of high school, I knew one thing for certain.

I couldn't stay the same and become the person I felt I needed to be.

For most of my childhood, I had felt out of place. I had spent years watching other people and wondering what they understood that I didn't. I had compared myself, questioned myself, and looked for some sign that I belonged.

Music was the exception.

When I played, especially when I stood onstage, I didn't have to ask myself where I belonged.

I knew.

There was something more out there for me. Something that felt connected to the person I became when I was playing music.

For the first time, the feeling of being out of place began to change.

It wasn't only an insecurity anymore.

It became a reason to leave.

CHAPTER THREE

Hollywood

"Welcome to the Jungle"
—Guns N' Roses

I left Ohio at eighteen years old with one clear idea in my head: I was going to become a rock and roll star. It didn't feel like some far-fetched dream or an idle fantasy. I believed it was real. It felt close enough to touch, like all I had to do was get myself to the right place and somehow the rest would begin to happen. In my mind, there was only one place I needed to be: Hollywood.

I was going to Musicians Institute, a school that was very direct about its mission. Guitar, bass, drums, vocals. Music. There were no distractions and none of the traditional college life I had never been interested in anyway. It offered a firsthand path into the world I thought I wanted, and that was enough for me. I didn't think much further than that. I didn't have some big plan or sit down and map out what success was supposed to look like or exactly how I was going to get there. I was eighteen years old. I wanted to play music, I wanted something bigger, and I knew I had to leave Ohio.

Life there had started to feel stagnant to me. I felt stuck. I had spent years trying to figure out where I belonged, and I was convinced that staying in the same place wasn't going to get me any closer to the answer. So I left. At eighteen, leaving home doesn't necessarily feel risky. It feels like freedom.

By the late 1980s, Hollywood had a very clear identity. The Sunset Strip had an energy that was difficult to ignore. It was exciting, electric, and dangerous all at the same time. Night after night, the clubs were filled with music. Bands and musicians were everywhere, and everybody seemed to be chasing something—fame, money, recognition, identity. It all blended together, and if you didn't know who you were when you got there, it was pretty easy to get lost in it.

I arrived with just enough confidence to believe I belonged and just enough insecurity to still feel like an outsider. My parents got me an apartment, and I was joined by two roommates. One was Dutch and named Vim. The other was French and named Stefan. We had come from different places, but we were all there for basically the same reason. We wanted to make music and leave some kind of mark in a city that didn't care whether any of us made it or not.

For the first time in my life, I was completely on my own. Nobody was watching me. Nobody was setting limits. Nobody was there to tell me what time to come home or what I should be doing with my day. School was the only real structure we had. That kind of freedom is exciting when you're eighteen, but freedom without much purpose or structure can become something else pretty quickly.

Musicians Institute was a wake-up call for me. Back in Ohio, I thought I was serious about music. I practiced. I rehearsed. I put in the time. I had taken summer school classes so I could make more room in my life for the band. I believed I understood what commitment looked like.

Then I got to L.A.

The level of talent hit me immediately. These musicians didn't just practice. They obsessed. They lived and breathed their instruments. Music wasn't something they did after everything else was finished. It was everything. They were technically skilled, but it went beyond that. They were disciplined in a way I had never seen before. They understood how to read music. They understood the business side of the industry. They thought about presentation, networking, and positioning themselves for opportunities. They approached music like a career long before it actually became one.

That was new to me. It wasn't that I lacked talent. I knew I had talent. The problem was that I wasn't nearly as prepared as I thought I was. I had come from a narrow background. Dublin, Ohio, had been my world for most of my childhood. It was where I grew up, went to school, formed a band, and started figuring out who I wanted to be. I didn't understand how big the world really was because I hadn't seen much of it yet.

Hollywood showed me, and Hollywood didn't ease you into anything.

I experienced things I had never seen before—violence, crime, addiction, desperation. None of it was hidden away somewhere. It was right there, part of everyday life. There were people chasing dreams everywhere you looked, but not everybody in Hollywood was running toward something. Some people were running from something. Others were already lost.

Being around all of it changed the way I saw the world. I wouldn't say it broke me. It didn't. But it pushed me further inward.

I had been in a relationship back in Ohio, and I tried to keep it going long distance. We tried to make it work, but it didn't last. When the relationship fell apart, it hit me harder than I expected. The emptiness I had felt in high school came back, only this time it felt stronger. Back in Ohio, I had my family. I had people who knew me and had known me for years. In Hollywood, I didn't have that same support system. I was eighteen years old, across the country, trying to become a rock star while still carrying around the same insecurities I had left Ohio with.

I didn't talk about any of it. I didn't open up to anyone and tell them how badly I was hurting. I didn't ask for help. That wasn't what I did. I shut it down because that was the only way I knew how to deal with it.

At first, nothing I was doing seemed like a problem. It felt like I was doing what everybody around me was doing. I had already been introduced to marijuana in high school. In Hollywood, it became more regular. It was accessible. It was normal. And it didn't stop there. Cocaine. LSD.

What started as experimentation became routine faster than I understood at the time. I didn't look at myself and think I was escaping from something. I didn't think I was coping with heartbreak or insecurity. I certainly wasn't using the words *self-medication*. I thought I was having fun. That's what people did in a place like L.A., right? At least, that's what I told myself.

Looking back, it's pretty obvious what was really happening. I was self-medicating. I just didn't know it yet. The noise in my head, the overthinking, the insecurity, and the constant questioning all became quieter when I was high. For a little while, I didn't feel inadequate. I didn't sit there wondering whether I belonged or comparing myself to the people around me. I got relief, and once you find something that gives you relief from your own head, it can become very easy to keep going back to it.

As strange as it sounds, I didn't feel as out of place in Hollywood as I had growing up. Somewhere in all the noise and chaos, I found a version of myself. I was in a couple of bands at the school. I performed regularly. People noticed my talent. There was validation, and for somebody who had spent most of his childhood questioning whether he was good enough, validation felt pretty damn good.

The problem was that it wasn't stable. It depended entirely on what was happening outside of me. When I played well, I felt good about myself. When people paid attention to me, I felt important. When somebody noticed my talent, I felt like maybe I really did belong there. When they didn't, I fell right back to where I had started. The same insecurity was still there. I had just found a louder place to hide it.

That cycle started taking hold of me. I began trying harder to stand out. I wanted to be louder. I wanted to be different. I thought maybe if I could get noticed, something would finally happen. At the time, I probably would have called that confidence or ambition. Looking back, it wasn't really confidence. It was a need to be seen.

That need hadn't started in Hollywood. It had been there since I was a kid. I had spent years wondering whether I was good enough, whether people liked me, and where I belonged. Now I was playing all of that out on a much bigger stage.

What I couldn't see at the time was that I wasn't usable in the way the music industry needed me to be. That's the truth. It had nothing to do with whether I had talent. It didn't even have anything to do with how motivated I believed I was. I wasn't consistent. I wasn't focused. I was distracted by everything around me.

The musicians who understood the business knew that talent was only part of it. You had to be disciplined. You had to be prepared. You had to show up and be someone other people could depend on. I had seen that level of commitment at Musicians Institute. I just wasn't living it myself.

Because of that, none of what I was doing turned into a real opportunity. I didn't understand that then. I thought I was doing what I was supposed to do. I thought the bands, the partying, the drugs, and the constant chase were all part of the process. I thought this was what becoming a rock star looked like.

Then a year flew by, and when it was over, reality hit me. I had no job. I had no gigs. I didn't even have a car. I skateboarded up and down Hollywood Boulevard every day, still trying to build something that didn't exist yet.

The dream hadn't disappeared. I still wanted to play music. I still believed there was something out there for me. But it wasn't working. At some point, belief runs into reality, and you have to look at where you actually are.

For me, that meant going back to Ohio. Not because I wanted to, but because I had to.

I didn't leave Hollywood feeling like a complete failure. It was more complicated than that. I had seen what it really took to succeed. I had been surrounded by musicians whose level of commitment, discipline, and sacrifice was unlike anything I had seen back home. I had learned that talent wasn't enough, even though I wasn't yet living by that lesson. I understood, at least on the surface, that music wasn't something you could take lightly if you expected to build a career from it.

That stayed with me, but other things stayed with me too: the habits, the coping mechanisms, the drugs, the way I shut things down instead of talking about them, and the urge to escape when being inside my own head became too much.

I didn't fully understand any of that when I left Hollywood. I didn't look at myself and see a problem. I thought I was doing the right thing by going home. I thought I had experience now, and in some ways, I did.

Hollywood had shown me how big the world was. It had shown me what serious musicianship looked like. It had shown me how much discipline it took to turn talent into a career. It had also introduced me to a way of dealing with pain that would stick around for years.

I carried both of those things back to Ohio with me.

I still didn't know what came next. I had no clear direction, and the version of the dream I had carried to Hollywood hadn't worked out the way I imagined. But I wasn't done with music. Not even close.

What I didn't realize yet was that the insecurity, the need to belong, being thrown into a world I wasn't ready for, and the way I had learned to deal with all of it were about to define everything that came next.

I had gone to Hollywood believing I would become a rock and roll star. I came home carrying something else.

I just didn't know yet how long I would carry it.

CHAPTER FOUR

Cowtown Nights

"I'm gonna live my life, can't stop for you, Gotta Keep a Runnin'"

SONG: GOTTA KEEP A RUNNIN'
BAND: THE GODZ

The late '80s and early '90s didn't arrive quietly. For me, they roared in with amplifiers, cigarette smoke, and the unshakable belief that if you were in a band, you mattered.

Columbus, Ohio, was alive in a way that's hard to replicate now. Around the Ohio State campus, bars weren't just places to drink—they were ecosystems. Every night carried the possibility of being discovered, or at the very least, being seen. The reality is that Columbus was barely a bug bite on the ass of the music industry. At the time, though, it didn't feel that way. To us, it felt like the center of the universe.

Live bands ruled our scene. If you had an instrument and could keep time, you had a place. Heavy metal was fading, grunge was creeping in, and somewhere in between there was room for anyone willing to get on stage and stay there long enough for something to happen. That's where I lived—not just geographically, but psychologically. I lived on stage, in bars, chasing the next set, the next reaction, and the next moment when the room turned toward me.

My first brush with anything resembling a record deal wasn't glamorous. There were no agents circling, no bidding wars, and no overnight success story waiting for me. I was nineteen years old, playing bass at an open jam session when a producer named Dave Egan noticed me. A small Columbus-based label called Sisapa Records had just started up, and Dave was producing a CD for a new artist they had signed, Karla Goldman. He invited me to audition.

I didn't get the gig.

At the time, I was working at a music store, and one of my coworkers was Mark Chatfield. Mark had played with Bob Seger and was a founding member of The Godz. More importantly to me, he was someone who had already been where I wanted to go. When I told him what had happened, he didn't sugarcoat anything. He told me exactly why I hadn't been hired.

My whole approach was wrong.

Mark suggested I get a Fender Precision Bass and even wired in new pickups for me himself. He told me to stop playing with my fingers and use a pick instead. He also told me to lower my strap so the bass hung around my waist instead of up by my chest like a jazz player. Looking back, those seem like small adjustments, but at nineteen they felt enormous. He wasn't just changing the way I played; he was teaching me how to present myself as a professional musician.

Then Mark did something I'll never forget.

He called the label himself and told them to give me another shot.

I went back with a completely different attitude.

This time, I got the gig.

That was the door opening.

My name was never on the deal, though. I wasn't the artist; I was part of the machinery behind it. I recorded the bass tracks and received writing credits on four songs, but eventually I was fired from the project. The label still pressed and released the CD, and my picture even appeared inside the jacket. The only problem was they had never finalized a publishing agreement with me before letting me go.

At that age, I only knew one way to respond.

I pushed back.

I leveraged whatever power I had and forced better terms. By then, I had already seen enough to realize the label wasn't planning to put much effort into promoting the CD anyway. In the end, I walked away with what I believed was a fair payout—probably more than they ever made back on the project itself.

There wasn't anything glamorous about the experience. No mythology. No fairy tale. It was simply my first real lesson that the music business was still a business.

After that, I joined a punk band called fronted by Mick Divens, with Mark on lead guitar. Playing alongside those two was electric. Mick already had independent releases circulating around the world, and before long we were opening for national acts like **Blue Öyster Cult** and **The Smithereens**.

Those shows fed my ego in ways I didn't fully understand at the time.

Every opening slot felt like proof that I was getting closer to the life I'd imagined. I wasn't just playing local bars anymore. I was sharing stages with bands I'd grown up listening to, and every opportunity convinced me I was moving in the right direction.

I stayed with **Boys From Nowhere** for about a year, and I'm still grateful for everything I learned from both Mark and Mick. They taught me far more than music. They taught me professionalism, stage presence, and what it looked like to take the business seriously.

Not long after that, I decided it was time to start my own band.

I called it **The Prayer**, then **The Final Prayer**.

Jeremy Rogers played drums, and Aaron Pauley played guitar. Both were incredibly talented musicians, and for the first time I wasn't helping someone else build a vision. This one was mine.

I wasn't planning on going to college, but my parents had helped all three of my brothers through school, and I think my dad realized that the path I had chosen was going to require support too—just in a different form. He believed in me enough to finance the production of our first CD.

We called it **The Doorway to America**.

I'm still grateful he did that.

The record turned out well, and before long we were being offered opportunities that had once seemed impossible. At one point we were invited to open for **Black Sabbath** in Columbus. For a young musician who had spent years dreaming about making it, that wasn't just another show—it felt like validation. More national opening slots followed, and every one of them reinforced the belief that maybe this was finally happening.

CDs became a kind of currency—not because they made money, but because they fed your ego. Releasing one felt like announcing your existence to the world. You told everyone you knew. You begged radio stations to play it. You asked bar owners to put it in their jukeboxes. Looking back, it all feels a little desperate, but at the time it felt like purpose.

The truth was there wasn't any real money in it. There was attention, and for me, attention had become its own reward. Long before I understood addiction, I had already become addicted to validation. Every compliment, every applause break, every opening slot, and every person who recognized my name fed something inside me that never seemed completely satisfied.

Eventually, disagreements within the band—and my own need for control—caught up with us. Jeremy and Aaron both left **The Final Prayer**, and I was forced to rebuild. Fortunately, Columbus was full of talented musicians, and over the next several years I rotated through different lineups, continuing to write, record, and perform whenever I had the chance. One of those bands even opened for **The Kinks**, another opportunity that seemed to confirm I was still moving forward.

On the surface, everything looked like progress.

Underneath, something very different was beginning to take shape.

The nights started to blur together. Performances turned into parties, and parties slowly became habits. Drinking wasn't something I did once in a while anymore—it had become part of the foundation of my life. More often than not, I was the last person sitting at the bar long after the music had stopped and most of the people had gone home. At some point, that stopped feeling unusual. It simply became normal.

I even moved into an apartment complex in Grandview that had its own bar inside the building. Looking back, that should have been a warning sign. Instead, I thought it was convenient. That's the funny thing about unhealthy patterns—they rarely announce themselves. They quietly settle into your routine until you stop questioning them.

Looking back now, I can see it wasn't just a lifestyle. It was avoidance.

I surrounded myself with people who drank the way I drank, lived the way I lived, and validated the way I avoided reality. They were good people. Some of them are sober today. Some aren't. Back then, though, none of us questioned much of anything. We simply accepted that this was the life musicians lived. As long as everyone around you is doing the same thing, it's remarkably easy to convince yourself there's no problem.

Emotionally, I was still a child.

Not in obvious ways. I could hold down a job, perform on stage, and handle responsibilities when I absolutely had to. But internally, I had no real framework for dealing with fear, rejection, disappointment, or uncertainty. Instead of confronting difficult emotions, I buried them beneath loud music, alcohol, late nights, and constant distraction. If I stayed busy enough, maybe I wouldn't have to deal with myself.

My relationships reflected that.

I met some incredible women during those years. Dawn, Kelly, and Alexandra would all remain important people in my life, although I had no way of knowing then how significant they would eventually become. At the time, they were simply part of the journey.

And then there were the others.

Some of the women I dated were professional go-go dancers and strippers. Some of those relationships lasted for a while. Most didn't. What always struck me wasn't the chaos people assume comes with that lifestyle, but the contradiction. They were kind, thoughtful, intelligent women who were often judged long before anyone bothered getting to know them. They often approached me, not the other way around. For a skinny guy with long hair playing in rock bands, that kind of attention felt like validation on a level I never questioned. They were beautiful, confident, and quite often they'd bring a girlfriend with them.

I always joke, "You can disappoint one woman in bed, but there's nothing like the feeling of disappointing two."

People laugh when I say that, and they're supposed to. Humor has always been one of the ways I've processed uncomfortable truths. Looking back, though, that joke says more about my insecurity than my confidence. I was still searching for validation in all the wrong places, convincing myself that attention meant fulfillment.

None of it was unique.

Ask any guy who played in a rock band during the late '80s or early '90s what life was like, and you'll probably hear a version of the same story. There was attention, access, and the illusion that somehow it would last forever.

It doesn't.

Slowly, another reality began settling in.

The record career I'd imagined wasn't materializing the way I'd hoped. I was still writing. I was still performing. I was still convinced the next opportunity might change everything. But years had gone by, and the breakthrough I kept expecting never came.

Then, in November of 1997, everything shifted.

One night, some friends and I walked into a dueling piano bar in downtown Columbus called Howl at the Moon. Two guys were on stage taking requests, joking with the crowd, and playing songs everybody knew. At first, I didn't really understand what made it different. It seemed entertaining enough, but I didn't immediately grasp why people loved it so much.

Then my friends threw twenty dollars on the piano, pushed me toward the stage, and told me to sing.

So I did.

I sang "Hey Jude."

When I finished, the general manager, Rich McClusky, and the entertainment director, Jed Demlow, pulled me aside and asked if I'd ever considered working there. I laughed and admitted I wasn't much of a piano player. They smiled and told me that wasn't really the point.

The job wasn't about being the best pianist in the room.

It was about being entertaining.

A few days later, I came back for a formal audition with Jed. Before long, I was working weekend happy-hour shifts and training under him.

To put it bluntly, I was a terrible student.

I questioned almost everything he told me. Every suggestion felt like criticism. I'd spent years fronting rock bands and opening for national acts, so somewhere in the back of my mind I believed I already knew how to entertain people.

I didn't.

The truth is, Jed was right about almost everything.

What I couldn't see then was the difference between performing for people and connecting with them. I knew how to stand on a stage and sing songs. Dueling pianos required something entirely different. It demanded interaction. You had to read the room, think on your feet, make people laugh, and make every customer feel like they were part of the show. The audience wasn't there to watch you perform. They were there to participate.

That lesson changed everything.

Jed wasn't the only one teaching me, either. Sunny Mullins, Jimmy Porter, Joe Laureano, and visiting player Todd Cutshaw all influenced the entertainer I would eventually become. Rich McClusky believed in me. Vice President Bob Dorko did too. Company founder Jimmy Bernstein, along with so many others at Howl at the Moon, helped shape my career in ways I'm still grateful for today.

I honestly owe my entire dueling piano career to that place.

For the first time in years, I had something I hadn't experienced before.

Structure.

I had regular work. A dependable paycheck. A place where people were genuinely invested in helping me improve instead of simply hoping I'd figure it out on my own.

Unfortunately, I also had something else.

Money.

And more money meant more opportunities to feed addictions I still wasn't ready to acknowledge.

Even years earlier, back in 1989, I'd had a frightening experience with mushrooms while working at a head shop. I needed counseling afterward. I went, but I wasn't ready to hear what anyone had to say. I stopped using drugs—for a while.

The drinking, however, never stopped.

Alcohol had become so woven into my life that I didn't even think of it as a problem anymore. It was simply what musicians did. We worked in bars, stayed out late, celebrated after shows, and drank with customers. It felt like part of the job description.

Then, in 1998, reality caught up with me. I was pulled over for drinking and driving. Looking back, it should have been the wake-up call I needed. Instead, it became another example of how addiction convinces you you're smarter than the consequences.

I knew enough about the legal system to keep my mouth shut. I refused the breath test. I refused the blood test. My driver's license was suspended for a year, but eventually the judge reduced the charge to reckless operation. At the time, I considered that a victory. Looking back now, I realize it wasn't a victory at all. It was another opportunity to change that I chose to ignore.

I didn't stop drinking.

I just started taking cabs.

That's the kind of logic addiction creates. Instead of fixing the real problem, you simply adjust your behavior enough to convince yourself you're being responsible. The drinking never changed. Only the transportation did.

By 2000, I was still writing and recording music whenever I could. No matter how much my life revolved around bars and dueling pianos, I never completely let go of the dream that had brought me to Hollywood years earlier. Somewhere inside me, I still believed music could become something more.

I submitted one of my songs, **"Into the Sun,"** to 99.7 The Blitz radio station for a local compilation CD. To my surprise, it was selected. It felt like another opportunity. Another reminder that maybe I wasn't finished chasing the dream after all.

My brother Sean believed in me enough to finance another project. We recorded a solo album under the name **B. Ryan Michaels**, a name I'd actually been using since the late 1980s. We hired producer Joe Viers, brought in professional musicians, found a manager, and even secured a promoter. For a while, it genuinely felt as though everything was lining up.

My single, **"Wild-n-Young,"** received airplay in different parts of the country. iTunes was just beginning to change the music industry, and we were among the early independent artists whose music was available on the platform. At the time, that felt significant. It felt like we were getting in on the ground floor of something that might finally open the right doors.

It still wasn't enough.

The record never became the breakthrough I'd spent years imagining. Eventually, Sean had to make the difficult decision to stop investing in the project.

That hurt more than I let anyone see.

It wasn't just because another dream had fallen short. It was because my brother had believed in me enough to put his own money behind my music. He wanted it to succeed every bit as much as I did, and despite everyone's efforts, we simply couldn't make it happen. My heart was broken for him.

Thankfully, I still had **Howl at the Moon**.

The job paid well. At that time, the room was full. Every weekend I was surrounded by music, laughter, and people who wanted to celebrate. From the outside, life probably looked pretty successful.

Underneath, the cracks were getting deeper.

The partying never really stopped. It just evolved. Drinking had become automatic, and before long, the drugs I thought I'd left behind started finding their way back into my life as well.

It didn't happen overnight.

It rarely does.

Addiction doesn't usually kick the front door down. It slips quietly back into your life until one day you realize it never really left.

Around the beginning of 2001, I started dating a nurse. She liked cocaine.

Just like that, I was back.

I wish I could tell you I fought it. I wish I could tell you I'd learned my lesson years earlier. The truth is, I didn't resist very much at all. It felt familiar. Comfortable. Normal.

Looking back, I understand what was really happening. Slowing down would have meant sitting alone with my thoughts, my disappointments, and the growing realization that the music career I'd imagined wasn't unfolding the way I'd planned.

I wasn't ready to face that reality.

So instead, I leaned in harder.

More shows.

More nights.

More drinking.

More noise.

As long as I stayed busy, I didn't have to think about what I was avoiding.

The nurse left...the habit stayed.

Then, something unexpected happened.

It wasn't the breakthrough I'd spent years chasing.

It was simply another opportunity.

The Columbus location of **Howl at the Moon** was beginning to slow down, and the company was preparing to open a brand-new location in Baltimore. Rich McClusky, the general manager who had believed in me from the beginning, was moving there to run it.

They needed players.

I needed work.

The opportunity couldn't have come at a better time.

When I looked at my life in Columbus, I realized I had quietly reached a crossroads. My record career wasn't becoming what I'd hoped. My addictions were becoming more difficult to ignore. Even though I didn't fully recognize it then, I think part of me knew I needed a change.

Baltimore represented exactly that.

A new city. A new stage. A new beginning. I wasn't moving because I had everything figured out. I was moving because standing still no longer felt like an option. Without spending much time overthinking it, I accepted the offer. At the time, I thought I was simply relocating for another job. Looking back now, I realize I was walking into one of the most important chapters of my life. I just had no idea how much it was going to cost me before it finally started giving something back.

CHAPTER FIVE

Baltimore

"I've been feeling so sick inside, got to better Lord before I die."

SONG: THE NEEDLE AND THE SPOON
Band: Lynyrd Skynyrd

The move to Baltimore in June 2001 wasn't driven by ambition as much as instinct. The Columbus location of **Howl at the Moon** was slowing down. You could feel it in the crowds, in the energy, and in the numbers nobody wanted to say out loud. At the same time, the company was preparing to open a new location in Baltimore, and my general manager, Rich McClusky, had been chosen to run it. They needed players. I needed work. So I packed up and went.

I wasn't arriving as a leader. I was simply another piano player helping open a brand-new venue in a city where I didn't know a single person. I had no expectations beyond doing my job, entertaining people, and figuring things out as I went. Within a few months, though, everything changed.

The entertainment director didn't show up one night.

There was no warning. No phone call. No explanation. He simply disappeared.

It happened on a Tuesday night, and suddenly I found myself carrying the entire show by myself. I played six straight hours with no rotation, no relief, and no backup. A fifty-seven-year-old customer who happened to know a handful of songs came up and helped me for a little while, but for the most part it was just me, two pianos, and a room full of people who still expected to be entertained.

The following day it became official.

The entertainment director wasn't coming back.

I saw an opportunity and picked up the phone. I called the company's vice president and told him I wanted the job. I wasn't interested in simply accepting more responsibility without the tools to succeed, so I negotiated. I wanted guaranteed money, and I wanted specific players brought to Baltimore—people I knew could help build a successful team. One of those people was Todd Cutshaw, who I considered one of the best entertainers in the business.

To the company's credit, they agreed.

Just like that, I wasn't simply performing anymore.

I was responsible for building something.

The problem was, I had no idea how to manage people.

The opening budget had already been stretched thin. The club was only about six months old, and financially it still wasn't stable. There wasn't enough money to keep flying experienced entertainers into Baltimore forever. We needed to build a local team, and we needed to do it quickly.

So I made a decision that, looking back, was probably one of the smartest decisions I'd made in my career.

I hired people who were better than me.

Some were veterans who already knew exactly how to run a room. Others were newer performers with the right attitude and enough talent to develop. My job wasn't to be the best player in the building. It was to put together a team that made the entire show better.

It worked.

Not perfectly, but well enough that we began building something we could all be proud of.

Outside the bar, however, life was much quieter.

I didn't know many people in Baltimore, and the staff gradually became my family. One family in particular took me in as though I'd known them for years.

Joan Gummer was a nurse. Her husband, Charlie, was one of the kindest men you'd ever meet, and their sons, Kevin and Jim—who bartended at the club—quickly became close friends. I spent weekends at their house, sharing meals, conversations, and a sense of normal family life I hadn't realized I'd been missing. Looking back, I can honestly say they gave me stability during a period when I desperately needed it.

For a while, it felt as though life was beginning to settle down.

Then everything started collapsing at once.

One night at the club, I was moving chairs when one slipped and crushed the ulnar nerve in my right arm.

At first, it was just pain.

Then my hand began going numb.

Eventually, it stopped working altogether.

For most people, an injured hand is an inconvenience.

For a piano player, it's an identity crisis.

Doctors prescribed pain medication, while physical therapists built me a device that looked like a claw so I could press basic chords on the piano. My right hand had lost nearly all of its dexterity. I wasn't really playing anymore. I was surviving.

But I kept performing.

Stopping never crossed my mind.

Then, just as I was trying to adapt to the injury, September 11, 2001 happened.

Baltimore wasn't New York, but it was close enough that everyone felt the impact. Many of our customers had friends, family members, or coworkers connected to the World Trade Center, the Pentagon, or the flights themselves. The entire country seemed frozen.

That day, we closed the club.

The following day, we reopened.

Management told us to keep people happy.

So we played.

The room filled with patriotic songs, and people openly cried while they sang. It quickly became obvious that we weren't just entertainers anymore. For many people walking through those doors, we had become part of the way they processed grief.

One night, a young woman in her early twenties sat beside me at the piano and requested **"American Pie."**

She told me her father and her boyfriend had both been in the towers.

She didn't know whether either of them was still alive.

She had no money to make the request.

I played it anyway.

She cried on my shoulder while I tried to smile through emotions I didn't fully understand myself.

Moments like that became common.

Grief wasn't something happening behind closed doors anymore. It was sitting right in front of us, asking for one more song.

Military personnel also became regulars at the club. We hosted send-off parties for men and women preparing to deploy overseas. Songs were dedicated to soldiers heading off to war. Then, months later, some of those same names returned—not for celebrations, but for memorials.

I started collecting the challenge coins they left on top of the piano.

Each one represented service, sacrifice, and a willingness to risk everything for someone else.

Looking at those coins, I couldn't shake a growing sense of guilt.

Here I was making nearly $150,000 a year playing music, leading a team, and entertaining crowds, while these men and women were preparing to leave for war.

It didn't seem fair.

I tried to compensate the only way I knew how. We organized care packages, collected donations, and did whatever we could to support the troops. Still, it never felt like enough.

While the country was changing around me, something else was changing inside me.

My injury wasn't improving.

The pain medication continued.

And without realizing it, I was about to cross a line I couldn't yet see.

While the country was changing around me, something else was changing inside me.

My arm wasn't healing the way I'd hoped. The pain lingered, and with it came prescriptions. At first, they were exactly what they were supposed to be—treatment. Doctors prescribed medication to help me function while my body recovered. But somewhere along the way, treatment quietly became dependency.

It didn't happen all at once.

The pain medication helped me get through the shows, and because I was still performing every night, it seemed justified. Then came Xanax to calm the anxiety that had always lived somewhere beneath the surface.

Alcohol had never left my life, and before long cocaine found its way back into the picture. Eventually, crack followed.

Looking back, I can see it wasn't one addiction replacing another. They simply stacked on top of each other until I could no longer tell where one ended and the next began.

Still, I performed.

That's what I knew how to do.

No matter what was happening in my personal life, I could walk onto a stage, smile, play songs people loved, and convince everyone—including myself—that everything was fine. Entertainment became both my profession and my disguise. As long as the audience was laughing and singing, nobody could see what was happening underneath.

The truth was, I didn't want them to.

If people believed I had everything together, then maybe I could believe it too.

Around early 2004, a group of younger people started coming into the club regularly. One of them was a beautiful young woman named Jennifer Doyle. Jenn was married, so there was never anything romantic between us. Nothing physical. We simply became friends.

It didn't take long for us to connect.

We talked on the phone often, and she and her friends continued coming into the club. Our conversations were easy. There wasn't any pressure to impress one another. We could simply talk, and over time I began trusting her in ways I hadn't expected.

Meanwhile, my addictions continued growing stronger.

I'd convinced myself they were simply part of the lifestyle. Everyone around me drank. Plenty of people used drugs. We worked late, entertained crowds, and lived inside an environment where excess didn't seem unusual. That became my justification.

As long as I wasn't the only one...

It couldn't really be a problem.

At least that's what I kept telling myself.

Then one night everything changed.

Jenn and I were talking on the phone when I suddenly passed out.

The next day I called her and asked what had happened. She told me I had started slurring my words before the conversation simply stopped. Hearing her describe it filled me with a kind of shame I hadn't experienced before.

I knew exactly what had happened.

I'd been drunk.

The words that immediately came into my mind weren't kind.

I thought I was a piece of shit.

I thought I was scum.

For the first time, I seriously wondered whether I could hide my addiction anymore.

What happened next surprised me.

Jenn didn't yell.

She didn't accuse me.

She didn't lecture me.

She didn't call me an alcoholic or a drug addict.

Instead, she quietly said something that completely disarmed me.

"You are sick."

Not broken.

Not weak.

Not a failure.

Sick.

She said it with genuine compassion.

Looking back now, I think that's exactly why it hit me so hard. If she had attacked me, I would have defended myself. If she had judged me, I would have dismissed everything she said.

Instead, she showed me empathy.

She saw me clearly...

and chose kindness anyway.

That did something to my ego I wasn't prepared for.

It hurt.

Because deep down, I already knew she was right.

She said it again: "You're sick," and followed it up with, "and you're gonna die just like me if you don't get help."

Jenn had been battling leukemia since before I'd met her.

If there had been a guaranteed treatment capable of curing her illness, she would have accepted it without hesitation. There would have been no pride. No denial. No excuses. She would have done whatever it took to live.

My situation was different.

The things standing between me and recovery wasn't just a disease I couldn't control.

It was me.

My pride.

My ego.

My refusal to admit that I no longer had control over my own life.

That realization didn't magically change everything overnight.

But it stayed with me.

It followed me.

Little by little, it wore down the walls I'd spent years building around myself.

Even then, I wasn't ready to surrender.

Instead, I kept trying to function as though nothing had changed.

I continued leading my team.

I continued performing.

I continued drinking.

I continued taking pills.

From the outside, life still looked manageable.

Inside, I was slowly collapsing.

Addiction has a remarkable ability to convince you that tomorrow will be the day you finally get things under control.

Tomorrow becomes next week.

Next week becomes next month.

Eventually, you stop making promises because even you don't believe them anymore.

That's where I was.

Still functioning.

Still performing.

Still pretending.

All while quietly moving toward the moment when pretending would no longer be possible.

By the summer of 2005, everything I'd spent years trying to hide had finally caught up with me.

I had been fired from Howl at the Moon for being late to a shift. On the surface, it seemed like a simple reason to lose a job. In reality, being late wasn't the problem. It was the symptom of a life that had completely spun out of control.

By then, my addictions were running every part of my day.

During the week, I was taking twelve to fifteen Norco pills at a time, along with six to eight milligrams of Xanax. That had become my normal. On weekends, I'd drink an entire handle of Jack Daniel's and smoke hundreds of dollars' worth of crack cocaine until Monday morning, when my body desperately needed pills just to function again.

The money wasn't steady anymore. The structure I'd built for myself in Baltimore wasn't enough to hold everything together. I was exhausted, buried in debt, and running on habits that weren't sustainable.

I had recently finished a run of shows in New Orleans, but they ended early because a hurricane was approaching. They sent me home on July 12.

Two days later...

I hit a wall.

There wasn't some dramatic Hollywood moment.

No audience.

No applause.

No one watching.

Just me.

Alone in my apartment.

I walked over to my red Lazy Boy chair, got down on my knees, and prayed with a level of honesty I'd never reached before.

"**God...** kill me or let me live. But I can't do this anymore."

There were no conditions.

No bargaining.

No promises.

Just complete surrender.

Almost immediately after I stood up, someone knocked on my door.

It was FedEx.

The package contained another shipment of pills.

Looking back, the timing still amazes me.

It felt like one final test.

I took the package inside and placed it on top of the refrigerator.

I didn't open it.

There was alcohol in the refrigerator.

There were drugs within arm's reach.

For the first time in years...

I left them alone.

I sat down and waited.

People often talk about detox as though it's simply feeling sick for a few days.

It isn't.

The first night was miserable.

The second morning was even worse.

I shook uncontrollably.

I sweated through my clothes.

I couldn't stop vomiting.

Diarrhea.

No sleep.

Every muscle in my body seemed to revolt against me.

By the second day, it felt as though my own body was trying to destroy itself.

Still...

I refused to touch the pills.

I refused to drink.

My friend Joan Gummer had already begun checking on me. As a nurse, she recognized what was happening long before I fully understood the danger myself. She kept calling, making sure I was still alive.

By the third day, it was obvious I wasn't okay.

I still refused to go to the hospital.

I thought I could simply tough it out.

I had no idea that withdrawing from benzodiazepines and opiates at the same time could actually kill me.

On the morning of July 17, I was barely functioning.

Joan couldn't force me to do anything, but she finally said something that got through to me.

"The doctors can give you drugs that will make this easier."

That was all I needed to hear.

Doctors.

Drugs.

Relief.

She helped me into her car and drove me to the hospital.

I remember trying to hold myself together during the drive.

The moment I walked through the hospital doors...

I completely lost it.

I threw up.

That day—July 17, 2005—is the day I consider my sobriety date.

Not because everything suddenly became better.

Not because the cravings disappeared.

But because it was the first day I stopped trying to treat myself...

and finally allowed someone else to help me.

That may not sound significant to most people.

For me, it changed everything.

I had spent my entire life believing I had to solve every problem on my own.

Asking for help felt like weakness.

Accepting help felt even harder.

For the first time in my life...

I surrendered.

The detox lasted several days.

Time blurred together into pain, exhaustion, confusion, and brief moments of clarity.

My family came.

Friends came.

People I hadn't expected showed up.

Then something happened that I've never forgotten.

The man visiting his father, who was sharing my hospital room, told me he had been sober for twenty years.

He asked if he could pray for me.

I said yes.

That moment stayed with me because it didn't feel accidental.

In fact, none of what happened during those days felt accidental.

One person after another seemed to appear exactly when I needed them.

Each conversation.

Each prayer.

Each act of kindness.

It felt as though God had been quietly placing people in my path all along.

The difference was...

for the first time...

I was finally willing to receive them.

After several days in the hospital, the doctors stabilized me. Their first priority was getting me safely through detox and making sure I wasn't in immediate danger. Looking back, I realize how close I had come. At the time, I simply knew I was exhausted. Physically, mentally, emotionally—I had nothing left.

I knew I needed treatment. My brother Sean's best friend at that time, Tom M, had been sober for quite some time and worked in recovery helping people find treatment facilities. He found just the right place for me. I do not believe any of this was coincidence.

Once I was medically stable, I was transferred to Cirque Lodge in Utah for treatment. I spent five days in the state hospital before entering the program, followed by thirty-one days at Cirque Lodge. For the first time in years, there were no bars to work in, no stages to perform on, no pills to numb me, and no alcohol to hide behind. There were no distractions left—only the truth.

Treatment wasn't about learning how to stop using drugs. It was about learning why I had needed them in the first place.

That was far more difficult.

For years, I had blamed my circumstances. The music business. Relationships. Stress. Success. Failure. Pain. Injury. There was always something outside of me that seemed responsible. Treatment forced me to look somewhere I had spent my entire life avoiding.

Myself.

It wasn't comfortable.

In fact, it was one of the hardest things I'd ever done.

I had spent decades building an identity around entertaining people, chasing approval, and trying to prove I was enough. When all of that was stripped away, I had to answer a question I'd never seriously asked before.

Who was I without the stage?

The answer didn't come quickly.

It came one conversation at a time.

One meeting at a time.

One day at a time.

By the time I completed treatment, one thing had become crystal clear.

Going back to the life I'd been living wasn't an option anymore.

My counselor told me about something I'd never heard of before—a sober living house in Los Angeles.

I asked him what a sober living house was.

He smiled and said, "It's a nice way of saying halfway house."

I agreed to go.

The decision surprised some people, but for me it made perfect sense. Los Angeles wasn't unfamiliar territory. I'd lived there once before as an eighteen-year-old chasing a rock-and-roll dream. This time, though, I wasn't going back to become a musician.

I was going back to learn how to live.

Before leaving, I spent two weeks at my parents' house in Ohio.

Those weeks were harder than I expected.

I had to sell nearly everything I owned.

Over the years, I'd collected guitars that weren't just instruments. They represented memories, milestones, and different seasons of my life. Together they were worth well over one hundred thousand dollars, but I sold them for only a fraction of that value.

I also sold my motorcycle to my best friend, Dennis.

None of those decisions were really about money.

They were about letting go.

Each item I sold felt like another piece of the identity I'd spent years constructing. Music had defined me for so long that I honestly didn't know who I would be without all the things I'd accumulated along the way.

I remember sitting on the floor in my parents' house, overwhelmed by a grief I couldn't fully explain.

I wasn't just mourning possessions.

I was mourning the version of myself that no longer existed.

Still...

I let it all go.

Because I knew I had to.

Eventually, the day came to leave for Los Angeles.

As I boarded the plane, I had no idea what waited for me. I wasn't chasing fame anymore. I wasn't chasing success. I was simply trying to stay alive.

Then something happened that, even today, I have trouble describing as coincidence.

The man sitting beside me asked why I was traveling to Los Angeles.

For perhaps the first time in my adult life, I answered honestly.

I told him everything.

When he heard my story, he smiled, switched seats with his wife, and introduced us.

She had been sober for decades.

We talked throughout the flight.

Looking back, it felt like another reminder that I wasn't walking this road alone.

Throughout my journey, people seemed to appear at exactly the right moment. Chris had been there when I needed medical guidance years later. Joan had helped save my life. Jenn had shown me compassion when shame couldn't. Now, on a flight to Los Angeles, I found myself sitting beside someone whose life had already become proof that long-term recovery was possible.

Another person.

Another conversation.

Another reminder.

By the time the plane landed, something inside me had begun to change.

Not dramatically.

Not all at once.

Quietly.

Hope had started replacing fear.

When I arrived in Los Angeles, people from the sober living house were waiting to pick me up.

Just like that, the Baltimore chapter of my life came to an end.

Everything I had built.

Everything I had accomplished.

Everything I had nearly destroyed.

It was behind me.

Not erased.

Not forgotten.

Simply finished.

Looking back now, I understand something I couldn't see then.

Baltimore gave me far more than a career.

It taught me leadership.

It taught me responsibility.

It introduced me to extraordinary friendships and people who would help save my life.

It also forced me to confront the consequences of years spent chasing validation while running from myself.

Without Baltimore, there would have been no collapse.

Without the collapse, there would have been no surrender.

And without surrender, there would have been no recovery.

For the first time in a very long time, I wasn't chasing applause.

I wasn't chasing another record deal.

I wasn't chasing another version of myself.

I was learning something much more important.

I was learning how to live.

I was learning how to stay sober.

And for the first time since I was a little boy trying to figure out where I belonged...

I was finally beginning to feel at home in my own skin.

CHAPTER SIX

Hollywood 2005

"Like a baby boy, I never was a man."

SONG: HATE ME
Band: Blue October

When I arrived in Los Angeles at the beginning of my sobriety, the city felt nothing like the Hollywood I'd experienced at eighteen. The first time I'd come here, I was driven by ego, fantasy, and adrenaline. I believed the city owed me something—that somewhere beneath the bright lights and crowded clubs, fame, validation, and identity were waiting for me. I came chasing a dream, convinced success would finally make me feel complete.

This time was different.

I wasn't carrying the illusion of becoming a rock star. I wasn't arriving with confidence or ambition. I wasn't even bringing the chemical buffer that had protected me from my own thoughts for so many years.

I arrived with a suitcase, a broken sense of self, and the uncomfortable realization that I had never really learned how to live.

That's the part people rarely talk about when they describe recovery. Most assume the hardest part is putting down the drink or the drugs. In my experience, it wasn't. The hardest part began after the substances were gone. That's when you're left standing alone with the same mind that drove you to them in the first place.

I was beginning to understand that if I wanted to stay sober, I would need something bigger than myself to rely on.

I moved into a sober living home called **Genesis House** on Los Angeles' west side. Eighteen other men lived there, all trying to do the same thing I was—stay sober one day at a time. The rooms were small. The bathrooms were shared. There were rules for everything: curfews, chores, meetings, accountability. Every day followed a structure.

Earlier in my life, I would have considered that environment suffocating. Back then, I believed freedom meant doing whatever I wanted, whenever I wanted. Looking back, I can see how wrong I was. My unstructured life had nearly killed me. I'd confused chaos with independence for years.

Real freedom isn't the absence of discipline.

Real freedom is living without fear.

Fear had quietly controlled my life for as long as I could remember. I'd been running from it since I was a little boy, even if I didn't have the words to describe it at the time. Whenever life became uncomfortable, I escaped into something else. Music. Attention. Relationships. Work. Alcohol. Pills. Cocaine. It didn't really matter what it was. If it distracted me from sitting alone with myself, I'd run toward it.

Now there was nowhere left to run.

No chemical escape.

No constant distraction.

Just silence.

And in that silence, everything I'd spent years avoiding finally caught up with me.

The first few months were emotionally brutal. It wasn't because I constantly wanted to get high. It was because I was finally forced to experience every emotion I'd spent years burying. Shame. Regret. Fear. Loneliness. Anxiety. Grief. Every feeling I'd numbed with alcohol, drugs, relationships, sex, shopping, dishonesty, and endless distraction came rushing back without any anesthesia.

Those things had worked for a while.

Then they became fun with problems.

Eventually, they were nothing but problems.

I had reached rock bottom.

Financially, I was bankrupt.

Spiritually, I was bankrupt.

Emotionally, I was exhausted.

At thirty-six years old, I had to admit something I never wanted to face.

I didn't have my life together.

For years I'd convinced myself I was functioning because I could still perform on stage, make people laugh, and earn a living. Underneath all of that, though, I'd never truly matured. I started getting loaded when I was sixteen, and emotionally I was still living from that same place. Instead of growing through life's painful experiences, I'd numbed them. Every time life demanded maturity, I'd found another way to run.

That realization hurt.

But it was also the first completely honest thing I'd admitted to myself in years.

And honesty became the foundation everything else was built upon.

One of the biggest misconceptions people have about recovery is that it's about humiliation—that you have to be broken down before you can rebuild yourself. That wasn't my experience at all.

Humiliation and humility aren't the same thing.

Humiliation tells you you're worthless.

Humility reminds you that you're not in control.

One destroys hope.

The other creates room for it.

Somewhere during those early months, I began sensing that something bigger than me might actually be capable of carrying what I never could.

For the first time in my life, I started surrendering.

I stopped trying to impress everyone around me.

I stopped pretending I had answers I didn't have.

Instead...

I listened.

Really listened.

The people around me came from completely different backgrounds. There were construction workers, executives, musicians, veterans, teachers, nurses, and doctors. On the surface, our lives couldn't have looked more different.

Underneath...

Our stories sounded remarkably alike.

Fear.

Shame.

Isolation.

That constant search for something outside ourselves that would finally make us feel okay.

Slowly, I realized something I had never believed before.

I wasn't uniquely broken.

For most of my life, I'd quietly carried the belief that everyone else had somehow received an instruction manual for life that I'd never been given. Sitting in those meetings shattered that illusion. Human beings are complicated. Most people are struggling with things nobody else can see.

Some are simply better at hiding it.

One of the first suggestions I received was to find a sponsor—someone who had already walked the path I was trying to follow. A sponsor wasn't there to solve my problems or tell me how to live every aspect of my life. Their role was to guide me through the recovery process, challenge my thinking, and help me stay accountable.

At first, I wasn't sure what I was looking for. I imagined someone gentle, endlessly patient, and full of comforting advice. Instead, I found myself meeting several temporary sponsors who all seemed convinced they knew exactly how my life should look. I was told to cut my hair, stay away from music, and find a quiet office job. None of that felt authentic to who I was. Sobriety wasn't supposed to erase my identity. I needed to learn how to live honestly, not become someone else.

Then one of my roommates at Genesis House, Mark, suggested I attend a meeting where his friend JT would be speaking. Mark knew the entertainment industry well. Before I met him, he'd worked on countless MTV videos throughout the late '80s and beyond. When he told me I should listen to JT, I trusted his judgment.

From the moment JT began speaking, something felt different.

He wasn't trying to impress anyone. He wasn't performing. He wasn't selling recovery or pretending life was perfect. He was simply comfortable in his own skin. There was a calmness about him that immediately caught my attention. As I listened to his story, I realized he'd accomplished many of the same things I'd spent years chasing—but he'd done them sober.

I wanted whatever that was.

After the meeting, I walked up and asked if he would sponsor me.

He looked at me and asked a simple question.

"Are you willing to go to any lengths to stay sober?"

I said "Yes".

It wasn't a confident answer. If I'm being honest, I probably mumbled it.

JT looked directly at me and said, "Don't waste my fucking time."

Oddly enough, it was exactly what I needed to hear.

There wasn't any cruelty in his voice. He wasn't trying to embarrass me or prove a point. He simply wanted honesty. He didn't care that I was a musician. He didn't care about my stories, my accomplishments, or my excuses. He cared about one thing: whether I was finally willing to tell the truth.

That conversation stayed with me.

People often quote the phrase, "The truth shall set you free."

What they don't usually mention is that the truth often hurts first.

One of the biggest revelations I had during those early months was realizing that alcohol and drugs had never actually been my problem.

They had been my solution.

The real problem was that I didn't know how to live peacefully inside my own mind.

That realization changed everything.

Recovery stopped being about resisting temptation. Instead, it became about creating a life I no longer wanted to escape from. The substances weren't the enemy. They were simply the symptom of something much deeper.

That process gradually became spiritual for me, although not in the way many people assume. Nobody handed me a religion. Nobody told me what I had to believe. What mattered was developing a relationship with something greater than my own ego—something greater than my fear, my need to control every outcome, and my endless attempts to manage life on my own terms.

For most of my life, I'd relied almost entirely on self-will. I believed that if I worked harder, controlled more, and avoided enough pain, I'd eventually figure everything out.

The truth was, self-will had landed me in a hospital bed.

I had run out of my own ideas.

For the first time, I became willing to try something different.

I had always believed in God, but believing in God and surrendering to God's will are two completely different things. Looking back, I had very little humility. Deep down, I still wanted life to unfold according to my plans. The idea that God's will might be different from what I wanted was something I struggled to accept.

Eventually, I reached a point where I had no choice but to become willing.

I started thinking about God in a way I'd never considered before. If God were small enough for me to completely understand, then God wouldn't be big enough to help me with the problems I couldn't solve myself.

That thought stayed with me.

I also began understanding that faith wasn't passive.

I could pray for food, but eventually I still had to get up, open the cupboard, or go earn the money to buy groceries. Prayer didn't replace action. It gave action purpose. I still had responsibilities. I still had to change the things I could change while learning to let go of the things I couldn't.

That balance became one of the most important lessons of my recovery.

Whatever fear I faced...

Whatever emptiness I felt...

Whatever challenges waited ahead...

I needed to place God between myself and those fears instead of trying to fight them alone.

That required honesty.

It required willingness.

And above all, it required fearlessness.

My sponsor encouraged me to begin taking a searching inventory of my life. Not just what I'd done, but why I'd done it. Why did I need approval so desperately? Why did rejection hurt me so deeply? Why was I terrified of being alone? Why did every achievement lose its meaning so quickly?

Those weren't easy questions.

But for the first time, I was willing to answer them honestly.

As I continued working through my inventory, I realized something I had spent most of my life trying to hide.

Beneath everything I'd accomplished, beneath the confidence I projected on stage, beneath the humor and the constant need to entertain, I was deeply insecure.

For years I had believed my greatest problem was addiction. Recovery taught me that addiction was only the symptom. The real issue was the way I saw myself.

I was carrying around enormous remorse, and during one of my conversations with my sponsor, he suggested that underneath much of it there were probably resentments. At first, I didn't understand what he meant. I didn't think of myself as an angry person. In fact, I was almost ashamed by the idea that I might have resentment toward anyone.

As I dug deeper, though, I realized my anger had never really disappeared.

I'd simply turned it inward.

Somewhere along the way, I'd convinced myself that what I thought didn't matter. What I felt didn't matter. In many ways, I had come to believe that my life didn't matter. Rather than standing up for myself, I spent years trying to avoid conflict at almost any cost. I walked on eggshells around people because I was terrified they wouldn't like me if I disappointed them.

I had never learned what healthy boundaries looked like.

Instead, I became whatever I thought other people wanted me to be.

Looking back, I can see how exhausting that was. My life had become one long performance, not just on stage, but everywhere. I hid behind dishonesty because I didn't believe the real me was enough. I wanted to feel nothing, because feeling anything seemed too dangerous.

When I looked honestly at the patterns that had shaped my life, one word kept appearing over and over again.

Fear.

Fear that I wasn't enough.

Fear that someone else would get what I wanted.

Fear that the girl I loved would leave.

Fear that she would be happy without me.

Fear of what other people thought.

Fear that if anyone truly knew me, they'd walk away.

Fear that unless I was performing, succeeding, entertaining, or receiving attention, I had no real value.

The more I examined those fears, the more I realized they all pointed toward the same thing.

Control.

I wanted to control how people saw me.

I wanted to control whether they stayed or left.

I wanted to control outcomes I had never been capable of controlling.

And because I couldn't...

my self-esteem disappeared.

That realization didn't magically fix my life.

But it helped me understand it.

Suddenly, years of addiction, unhealthy relationships, workaholism, perfectionism, and the constant search for validation all made sense. They weren't separate problems.

They were different expressions of the same wound.

For the first time, I stopped trying to earn my worth and began considering the possibility that maybe my worth had never depended on performance in the first place.

That thought softened something inside me.

I became less defensive.

Less reactive.

Less concerned with proving myself every time I walked into a room.

Recovery taught me something wonderfully simple.

Esteemable acts build self-esteem.

Not applause.

Not compliments.

Not record deals.

Not money.

Doing the next right thing.

Keeping my word.

Showing up.

Living honestly.

That's how self-respect begins.

As I continued working with my sponsor, I shared things I'd never admitted out loud before. Years of fear. Shame. Pride. Dishonesty. Sexual history. The more I talked, the lighter I felt. It was as though I had spent decades carrying a backpack full of rocks without realizing I could simply set it down.

Little by little, I started becoming comfortable in my own skin.

Not because I'd become perfect.

Because I had finally stopped pretending.

Life continued moving while all of this was happening.

Jennifer and I remained in close contact throughout my time at Genesis House. We talked almost every day, and every conversation reminded me of the extraordinary grace she carried despite everything she was facing. She had every reason to become bitter, angry, or resentful. Instead, she chose compassion.

I couldn't stop comparing her strength to my own life.

I'd been given countless opportunities and nearly thrown them all away.

She had been handed circumstances no one would ever choose, yet somehow continued treating people with kindness.

That contrast stayed with me every single day.

Then one morning, I called her as I usually did.

Someone else answered the phone.

Jennifer had passed.

I had one hundred days sober.

The news hit me in a way I wasn't prepared for.

Sometimes life doesn't stop when someone dies.

It simply rearranges itself.

I remember feeling grief, gratitude, guilt, and clarity all at the same time. Jennifer had seen something in me before I was capable of seeing it in myself. She never treated me as though I were broken beyond repair. She simply saw someone who had lost his way.

Instead of judging me...

she loved me with compassion.

That compassion became one of the reasons I'm alive today.

After Jennifer died, I had a vision.

She was standing peacefully beside a white tiger.

There was no fear.

No sadness.

Only peace.

People can interpret experiences like that however they choose. Maybe it was grief. Maybe it was my subconscious trying to process loss. Maybe it was something I can't explain.

The explanation matters less to me than the feeling it left behind.

Peace.

For the first time in a very long time, I began believing that peace wasn't something reserved for other people.

Maybe...

it was possible for me too.

Genesis House allowed me to return to Baltimore for Jennifer's funeral.

Joan Gummer picked me up at the airport, and once again the Gummer family welcomed me into their home as though I were one of their own. Being back in Baltimore felt strange. It was a city filled with memories—some wonderful, many painful. Walking through those familiar places, I realized just how much my life had changed in a relatively short period of time.

At Jennifer's funeral, I had the opportunity to speak with her parents. I told them what Jennifer had meant to me and how profoundly her compassion had influenced my recovery. I wanted them to know that their daughter had done far more than offer friendship. She had helped save a life.

They listened with extraordinary kindness.

Before we parted, they told me I could call them anytime.

For reasons I couldn't fully explain then, I didn't feel as though that would be the last time our lives would intersect.

Returning to Los Angeles meant returning to accountability.

One of the rules at Genesis House was simple: if you left town, you were urine tested when you came back. Shortly after returning from Baltimore, I provided a urine sample. Had I used drugs or alcohol while I was away, I would have been asked to leave the house immediately.

I wasn't worried.

For the first time in my adult life, I genuinely wanted to stay sober.

The test came back clean.

It wasn't simply a matter of passing a drug test.

It was evidence that something inside me had begun to change.

Recovery wasn't just becoming something I talked about.

It was becoming the way I lived.

I continued working closely with my sponsor, attending meetings, and slowly making amends to the people I had harmed. Before recovery, I thought an amends was simply another word for an apology. I eventually learned it was much deeper than that.

Making amends meant honestly acknowledging my part in the damage I'd caused, understanding why I had behaved the way I did, and doing whatever I reasonably could to repair that harm. It also meant resisting the temptation to point out someone else's mistakes. Recovery taught me to focus on my own side of the street before worrying about anyone else's.

That lesson wasn't easy.

For most of my life, I'd been far more comfortable explaining why other people had contributed to my problems than honestly examining the role I'd played in creating them.

Accountability changed that.

Somewhere around my 7th month of sobriety, something happened that I never imagined would happen so soon.

I took on my first sponsee.

It felt surreal.

Only months earlier, I had been fighting for my own life. Now someone else was asking me to help them begin their recovery. I wasn't an expert. I certainly didn't have everything figured out. But I'd been freely given something by the people who had helped me, and part of recovery is passing that gift along.

I began to understand that helping someone else stay sober strengthened my own sobriety as well.

For the first time in my life, I genuinely felt that God was working through me instead of simply working around me.

Life slowly became less dramatic.

That may not sound exciting, but after years of living in constant chaos, ordinary life became one of the greatest gifts I'd ever received.

I started working again.

I started playing music again.

I showed up on time.

I kept my commitments.

I did the small, ordinary things that most people take for granted.

For me, those things represented enormous victories.

After years of being unreliable, I was becoming someone others could depend on.

After years of hiding behind excuses, I was learning accountability.

After years of avoiding eye contact because I always had something to hide, I could finally look people in the eye without feeling ashamed.

There was something deeply humbling about that process.

Humility didn't make me think less of myself.

It helped me think less about myself.

I no longer felt the need to control every conversation, every room, or every outcome. I wasn't doing it perfectly—far from it—but I was trying. That alone represented a tremendous shift from the person I'd been only months earlier.

Without fully realizing it, I was changing.

Not into someone new.

Into someone more honest.

I was still emotional.

Still insecure at times.

Still imperfect.

But I was no longer running from every uncomfortable feeling that entered my life.

Eventually, another opportunity presented itself.

Music began calling me back.

Part of me was excited.

Another part was terrified.

For most of my life, music had been inseparable from my ego, my addictions, and my desperate need for validation. The stage had been where

I searched for approval, escaped from myself, and built an identity that couldn't survive once the applause stopped.

Now I had to answer a different question.

Could I return to music without losing myself again?

The answer wasn't obvious.

There was also a practical reality I couldn't ignore.

Around three months into sober living, I had filed for bankruptcy. I had almost nothing left financially. A wonderful organization called MusiCares had been paying my rent at Genesis House while I focused on rebuilding my life. Their generosity gave me the time I desperately needed to recover without immediately worrying about where I was going to sleep.

When my counselor at Musicares, Shireen, told me months before that they could help me, I broke down in tears in her office. I wanted to stay sober, and she could see that.

But now it was time.

Time for me to begin supporting myself again.

Time to become responsible for my own life.

I knew I needed to work.

I knew I needed to become financially independent.

And I knew that sooner or later, music would become part of that journey again.

This time, however, it couldn't be about ego.

It couldn't be about proving myself.

It couldn't be about chasing validation.

If I was going back, it had to be different.

It had to come from a healthier place.

The truth was...

I didn't know whether that was possible.

But I was beginning to trust something I had resisted for most of my life.

I didn't have to know every answer before taking the next step.

God did.

And, as they say in recovery...

More would be revealed.

CHAPTER SEVEN

Returning to the World

"I Can't stand this indecision, married with a lack of vision"

SONG: EVERYBODY WANTS TO RULE THE WORLD
BAND: TEARS FOR FEARS

By April 2006, I had reached the point sober living had been preparing me for. I had to leave Genesis House and find out whether anything I had learned there would follow me into the outside world.

Genesis House had given me structure when I was incapable of creating any for myself. There had been rules, chores, curfews, meetings, drug tests, and eighteen other men trying to remain sober under the same roof. The structure had felt restrictive when I first arrived, but over time, it became one of the things keeping me alive. Now I would have to live without anyone standing nearby to enforce it.

I moved into a small garage apartment with my friend Brian, whom I knew from sober living. Brian had a girlfriend and was rarely at the apartment, so most of the time I was there alone. That was a significant change after living in a house where privacy barely existed, and someone was always aware of what I was doing.

At Genesis House, there had always been people asking where I was going, when I was coming back, and whether I had done what I said I would do. I might have resented those questions at times, but I could not pretend nobody was paying attention. In the garage apartment, nobody was watching. There was no house manager, no curfew, and no mandatory schedule posted somewhere for me to follow.

I had wanted freedom for most of my life, but now that I finally had some, it made me nervous. Freedom itself had never been my problem. What I did with it had been the problem.

I was still attending recovery meetings, working with my sponsor, and praying on my knees at night. I had also begun taking other people through the same work that had been freely given to me. Those things provided a foundation, but they did not pay rent, and the practical responsibilities of life had not disappeared just because I had become sober.

A few months into sober living, I had filed for bankruptcy. Financially, there was very little left. I was grateful to be alive, but gratitude did not remove the bills waiting for me outside Genesis House. I needed to support myself again, and the most obvious place to look was also one of the places that frightened me most: music.

For nearly my entire life, music had been where I felt most comfortable. It had also become connected to nearly everything that had destroyed me. Bars, alcohol, drugs, attention, ego, late nights, applause, and the constant need to be seen had all become tangled together with performing. Returning to music meant returning to the same environment where much of that destruction had developed.

At the same time, music was the one professional skill I had. I could not pretend that part of my life had never existed, and I did not yet know what else I was qualified to do. Eventually, I called Howl at the Moon and begged them to let me come back.

Howl at the Moon had given me my dueling-piano career. The company had trained me, trusted me, and eventually placed me in leadership positions. I had also taken those opportunities and nearly destroyed myself while holding them. They did not owe me another chance, but somehow, I received one anyway.

I began working at the Hollywood location while I was still living at Genesis House. Three or four nights a week gave me regular income and something productive to do. By the time I moved into the garage apartment, I had already started rebuilding a work routine, and showing up sober felt different from anything I had done before.

Before recovery, I often believed that simply arriving for work meant I was doing my job. It did not matter what condition I was in, how much I had used the night before, or whether the people around me had to compensate for my behavior. If I got onstage and made it through the show, I considered myself reliable.

Now reliability meant something else. It meant arriving on time, being prepared, keeping my commitments even when nobody praised me for doing it, and leaving at the end of the night without using anything. Those were basic expectations, but after years of living the way I had, ordinary responsibility felt like a major accomplishment.

The stage itself had not changed, but parts of me had. Other parts were still catching up, and that became obvious very quickly.

I had spent years in leadership positions and was accustomed to being the entertainment director, making decisions, controlling the stage, and telling other performers what needed to happen. Returning to Howl at the Moon meant returning as an employee rather than the person in charge. I told myself I was grateful for the opportunity, and I truly was, but I also had opinions about almost everything.

One of the strange things about early sobriety is that once your mind starts clearing, you can suddenly become very confident about everything you think. You have spent months examining your life, learning new ideas, and discovering a different way to live. It can make you believe everyone needs to hear what you have recently learned.

They do not. Not every thought needs to become a speech, not every disagreement requires your intervention, and not every workplace decision needs your approval. I had not learned that yet.

I was sober, but I was still uncomfortable when I was not the decision-maker. I had spent most of my life trying to control people and situations because control made me feel safe. Removing drugs and alcohol had not removed that instinct. It had only made it easier to see.

While I was working at Howl, another musical opportunity appeared. I was asked to audition for a children's country-music group called the Bumkin Band.

Country music for kids was not exactly the direction anyone might have predicted for me. My background was rock, punk, dueling pianos, and late-night bars. I had spent years performing for adults who were drinking and requesting the same songs at increasingly louder volumes. The Bumkin Band was something completely different, and that was part of what made it special.

The group included Kimber Breaux and Sam Nickel. Kimber was a gifted lyricist who wrote children's songs with humor, warmth, and intelligence. By the time I met her, she had seventeen years of sobriety, while I was not even a year into mine.

Kimber became an important person in my life because she understood both parts of me: the musician and the person trying to live sober. I did not have to explain why returning to music could feel exciting and dangerous at the same time. She had already proved that a creative life and a sober life did not have to destroy each other.

For years, I had associated making music with chaos, but Kimber showed me another possibility. The three of us wrote enough music for an entire record, performed at the first two Stagecoach Festivals in 2007 and 2008, and also appeared at the Austin City Limits Music Festival.

Those were significant stages, but the emotional experience was different from the performances I had chased earlier in my life. I was not standing there trying to prove I was a rock star. I was participating in something designed to make children and families happy. There was no need for darkness behind it, and there were no drugs, alcohol, or self-destruction required.

It was music without the same baggage. That did not mean I had suddenly become easy to work with everywhere else.

After approximately six months back at Howl at the Moon, I was fired. I could have blamed personalities, management, politics, or any number of outside factors. Earlier in my life, I would have built an entire case explaining why everyone else was wrong, and to some extent, I did, but the truth was simpler.

I still did not know how to stop trying to run everything. My opinions had returned before my humility was fully developed. I had started believing that because I was sober and working on myself, I knew what should happen around me. Not everyone wanted to hear what I thought, and the easiest solution for the company was to remove me.

Being fired hurt, but it also forced me into a larger professional world. Without a regular Howl position, I began traveling nationally to perform at other dueling-piano venues. I flew out on weekends and worked with players in different cities, each of whom had a different catalog, style, and method of controlling an audience.

The traveling expanded my professional network, but it also exposed me to something I had never handled well: other people's talent. When you are deeply insecure, another person's talent does not always look like an opportunity to learn. Sometimes it looks like a threat.

I had spent years measuring myself against everyone around me. I noticed who could sing higher, who knew more songs, who received more applause, who was offered the position I wanted, and who was making more money. Sobriety did not immediately shut off that part of my mind. It gave me a chance to notice it, and there was a difference.

During 2007, I worked in Las Vegas frequently. At the end of that year, I met a woman I'll call T, and we fell deeply in love.

Through 2008, I traveled back and forth to Las Vegas to work and spend time with her. For a while, the relationship brought warmth and excitement into a life that had been dominated by recovery and rebuilding. I wanted love, but the problem was that I had spent most of my adult life confusing love with emotional rescue.

I wanted another person to make me feel secure. I wanted reassurance that I was enough, and I wanted closeness without understanding how to tolerate uncertainty, conflict, distance, or the possibility of rejection.

I had stopped using drugs and alcohol at thirty-six years old, but emotionally, parts of me were much younger. For roughly twenty years, every time an uncomfortable emotion appeared, I had numbed it. I did not process heartbreak, insecurity, jealousy, fear, or abandonment in a healthy way. I escaped them.

When you spend decades avoiding emotions, you do not mature simply because you finally stop using them. You still have to feel everything you avoided, and you still have to learn what to do with it.

T and I loved each other, but love alone could not correct all of that emotional immaturity. Eventually, the relationship ended, and I was devastated.

I would like to say I accepted the loss with grace because I was sober and spiritually grounded, but I did not. I was heartbroken, angry, resentful, and wrecked. The difference was that I did not use.

That may not sound like enough, but at that stage of my life, it was enormous. For most of my adult life, pain had been followed by escape. If a relationship ended, I drank. If rejection hurt, I used. If I felt abandoned, I found something that would make me feel nothing. This time, I had to experience the loss while remaining present for it.

I talked about it, went to meetings, called people, prayed, and continued working. None of those things made the heartbreak disappear immediately. Recovery did not make pain painless. It gave me a way to survive pain without turning it into another catastrophe.

T would eventually return to my life in another way, but at that point, I had to keep moving, and by 2008, I had secured a regular house gig at Sergeant Peppers in Long Beach.

The job gave me steady work, which I needed, but it also required a brutal commute from Hollywood. Depending on traffic, getting to Long Beach could take two or three hours, and coming home could take another one to three. I was working five nights a week, and although I was grateful for the job, I was exhausted.

Los Angeles traffic can turn a relatively simple distance into half of your day. I spent hours sitting in a vehicle, worked late into the night, and then made the same trip again. Still, I kept showing up.

One night, another piano player from Los Angeles came into Sergeant Peppers and sat in for a song. His name was Donny Scott, and the moment he started singing, fear went through me.

Donny was one of the greatest singers I had ever heard on a dueling-piano stage. His voice was powerful, his range was extraordinary, and his presence was immediate. My first thought was not that he was incredible. My first thought was that he had come to take my job.

That was how insecurity still worked inside me. Another person could walk into a room, do something well, and before I knew anything about his intentions, I had already imagined myself being replaced.

Donny was not there to take my job, and he was not secretly auditioning for my position. He sat in, performed the song, and left an impression on me that stayed long after the night ended.

I remember thinking that if I ever had a place of my own, I needed to find him. At the time, I did not know what that place would be, and I certainly did not know that Donny would eventually become one of the most important people in my life. I only knew what I had heard: the guy could sing his ass off.

Not long afterward, an opportunity opened in Claremont, California. A piano bar called Piano Piano was being built as part of a hotel, and they needed an entertainment director.

The position appeared to offer nearly everything I thought I wanted. It came with health insurance, allowed me to stay at the hotel when necessary, and offered the highest salary I had ever received. After years of instability, bankruptcy, sober living, and trying to rebuild my life one commitment at a time, the opportunity looked like security.

I left Sergeant Peppers and accepted the position. By then, I had been sober for a little more than three years. I was still living in Hollywood and attending recovery meetings there, but I spent four or five nights a week at the hotel in Claremont.

My responsibility was to build the show. I had done this before, knew how to develop performers and structure a night, and had worked under some of the people who helped create the modern dueling-piano format. I understood the traditions of the business and the rules that had been passed down to me.

I also knew how difficult opening a piano bar could be. Everyone has an opinion when a venue is struggling to find its identity. Managers, hotel executives, food-and-beverage departments, employees standing near the stage, and customers all believe they know what the show needs.

Most of those people cannot sit down at the piano and carry the performance, but they can still tell you exactly how they believe it should be done. That became one of the most frustrating parts of opening Piano Piano. There were too many voices with zero experience.

The difference between Claremont and Baltimore was that I was now sober enough to recognize the dysfunction while it was happening. Unfortunately, recognizing dysfunction does not automatically mean you know how to respond to it. Sometimes it simply means you're more conscious of how angry it makes you.

I was still early enough in recovery that I wanted to tell everyone how I saw the world. When you first discover a spiritual way of living, you can become overly enthusiastic about sharing it. You start seeing dysfunction, addiction, dishonesty, and ego everywhere.

Sometimes you're seeing those things accurately. At other times, you're using your new awareness as another reason to judge people, and I had to learn the difference.

I also had to learn that I could not become the sobriety police for everyone around me. I worked in a bar where people drank. Some drank more than I thought they should, and some behaved in ways I recognized from my own past. That did not make their lives my responsibility. My responsibility was my own behavior.

When I began building the Claremont team, I remembered Donny. I contacted him and asked whether he would come work with me.

Donny had already made a commitment to help open another piano bar later, so he could not remain permanently. He agreed, however, to work with me for approximately three months and help get Piano Piano started. Those three months changed the way I looked at the show.

Donny brought ideas I had never seen before. He used props, introduced bits, and found ways to interact with the audience that did not fit neatly inside the rules I had been taught. My immediate reaction was resistance because I believed those things were not how the show was supposed to work.

I had learned from some of the most respected people in the dueling-piano industry and believed there was a correct way to build the performance. Anything outside that structure initially looked wrong to me. Recovery, however, had taught me that my first thought did not always have to become my final decision, so I kept my mouth shut long enough to watch.

The audience loved what Donny was doing. They were not concerned that he had broken an unwritten rule I had learned years earlier, and they did not care whether a bit had been approved by the traditional dueling-piano establishment. They were laughing, singing, participating, and having a great time. That was the job.

I had to admit that Donny was doing things I could learn from, and that admission represented more growth than it might appear. Earlier in my life, I would have felt threatened. I might have shut down his ideas simply because they had not come from me, using my position to protect my authority instead of improving the show.

This time, I watched the audience. Donny could also sing songs I could not sing, and his voice opened possibilities for the performance that my voice did not. Instead of treating that as proof that I was inadequate, I slowly began understanding what a real partnership could look like.

He did not need to be less talented for me to remain valuable. His strengths did not erase mine, and together, we could create something neither of us could create alone.

The partnership became incredible, but I knew Donny had already made another commitment and would eventually leave. I had accepted that from the beginning, although knowing it did not make his departure easy.

By then, I understood how rare it was to find someone whose talent challenged me while his presence made the entire show better. I wanted him to stay, but he had given his word elsewhere, so he left. Through Donny, I also met Steve Haas, another exceptional performer who had worked with him at a previous venue. That connection would matter later.

At Piano Piano, other players came and went. Some relationships worked, and others did not. Meanwhile, my relationship with the hotel management continued deteriorating.

I did not feel supported, and management did not always appreciate the way I communicated. I believed I was being asked to carry responsibility without being given the freedom to make the decisions necessary for the show to succeed.

Eventually, I was called into an office in front of several managers and instructed to apologize to the head of housekeeping, who believed I had been rude to him. I thought the entire situation was bullshit, and some of the managers privately told me they agreed with my side. That did not change what I was being required to do.

I made the apology. Recovery had taught me to examine my part in conflict, but it had also taught me that apologizing did not always mean agreeing with every version of an event. Sometimes it meant acknowledging that the way I communicated had caused harm, whether I intended it or not.

I tried to practice that, but I would be lying if I said I walked out of the meeting filled with spiritual peace. I was resentful. I hated being brought into a room and made to apologize in front of a group of managers, and I hated feeling that people who did not understand the show could interfere with how I was trying to run it.

That was when I started telling myself I never wanted to be part of another business with a human-resources department. It was probably not the most balanced conclusion, but it was honest.

The environment had become unhealthy for me. I was spending most of the week away from home, surrounded by workplace conflict, and becoming increasingly frustrated by the number of people involved in every decision.

I also felt awkward being the sober person in an environment where many people drank. I did not want to lecture anyone or become the wet blanket in the room, but I could no longer ignore certain behaviors in the way I once had. Sobriety had changed what I could tolerate.

Still, not everything about Claremont was negative. I met extraordinary people in the audience, some of whom became lifelong friends. Several would later appear when I faced situations far more serious than workplace politics, although at the time, I could not have known that. I only knew they continued showing up to hear us play.

During that period, I began accepting a small number of private events on my own. I had no real company structure behind them and was simply testing the idea that dueling pianos could exist outside a permanent bar.

In 2009, I created a name for those shows: The Killer Dueling Pianos. I also started a Facebook page under that name.

That was the entire company. There was no logo, website, professional video, large roster, or established client base. There was only a name, a Facebook page, a few private events, and a thought beginning to form in my mind.

At that point, Piano Piano was still paying me extremely well. I was earning a couple hundred thousand dollars a year with benefits, and walking away from that kind of money seemed irresponsible. Staying, however, was making me miserable.

Another piano bar was preparing to open in Fullerton. It was called Zings, and the owners had been encouraging me to join them. The position would pay approximately fifty-five thousand dollars a year with no benefits. It was not a small pay cut; it was almost a financial demolition.

I was ready to quit Piano Piano immediately, but my sponsor stopped me and told me to write an inventory. In recovery, an inventory is not simply a list of complaints. It is an honest examination of the situation, including your own motives, fears, resentments, and responsibilities.

He told me to list everything I hated about the job and then write down everything I would miss. When I finished, the answer became obvious. The only thing I was going to miss was the money.

My sponsor reminded me that I had made a couple hundred thousand dollars a year in Baltimore and had still been unable to stay sober. "The money isn't going to fix you," he told me.

He was right. Money had never been the real problem. The absence of it frightened me, but having it had not made me peaceful, created self-respect, healed my insecurity, or made me emotionally mature. It certainly had not kept me sober.

I tried to leave Claremont with a clean conscience. I practised forgiveness where I could, made amends where I believed I owed them, and reminded myself that nobody else was responsible for how I chose to respond.

Some of the people there had been wonderful, while others had been extremely difficult for me. In the end, I was still responsible for myself.

That did not mean I left without resentment, because I did, but recovery did not make me incapable of resentment. It gave me a process for recognizing it before it destroyed me.

I accepted the position in Fullerton. Almost immediately, many of the promises surrounding the new venue began disappearing.

There had been talk of promotion and building something significant, but once I arrived, much of that energy seemed to vanish. The owners reduced their promotional efforts and nearly abandoned the larger vision for the piano bar.

My responsibilities, however, were much lighter. I no longer had to manage an entire hotel operation's expectations or remain on-site for most of the week. For the most part, I needed to show up four nights a week and perform. The money was dramatically lower, but so was the pressure.

I moved into a house in Claremont with a musician friend who was renting it. That shortened the drive to Fullerton and allowed me to leave Hollywood behind.

The Fullerton room was rarely full, and this was not a glory gig. There were no massive crowds waiting outside and no sense that we had become the center of Southern California nightlife. Some nights, we were trying to create energy in a room that offered very little back, but we still had to perform.

A nearly empty room can expose an entertainer in ways a packed room does not. When hundreds of people are singing, their energy carries you. When only a few people are watching, you have to generate that energy yourself because you cannot hide behind the crowd.

We needed another full-time player. A few years earlier, in 2007, I had visited a piano bar in Phoenix and met a performer named Johnny Greco.

Johnny was approximately five-foot-six, but his energy was enormous. He was physically explosive onstage, an outstanding musician, and capable of delivering songs in ways I had never seen. His catalog was also incredibly broad.

By the time I was working in Fullerton, Johnny was looking for a full-time position in California. We reconnected, and he came aboard.

Johnny and I clashed at first, which was not unusual for me. We had different strengths, different instincts, and different ideas about certain parts of the show. I had been working in dueling pianos for years and carried strong opinions about how things should be done. Johnny had strong opinions too.

He could also do things I could not. He knew songs I did not know, approached performances in ways I never would have considered, and brought an energy that forced me to expand my understanding of what the show could be.

The same thing had happened with Donny, and a pattern was developing. The people who challenged my ideas were often the same people who helped me grow.

For years, I had believed leadership meant having the answers. I was beginning to see that leadership might mean bringing in people whose answers were different from mine.

Johnny and I learned from each other. We played four nights a week in a room that was rarely full and continued giving the people who did show up the best performance we could. We slugged it out together, and there was value in that.

Not every stage in a career is glamorous. Some are simply where you develop the endurance and relationships you will need later.

Private work continued arriving occasionally under The Killer Dueling Pianos name, but not much. There might be one show followed by another opportunity somewhere else, yet nothing about it looked like a real business.

I was still relying on someone else's venue for most of my income, working inside another person's vision, and learning what I liked and disliked about the way entertainment businesses were managed. Even so, something was changing.

At Howl at the Moon, I had been given a system. At Piano Piano, I had been given authority and money, along with dysfunction I could not control. At Ziings, I had less authority, much less money, and fewer expectations. Each place was teaching me something.

Howl taught me the craft. Claremont taught me what happened when too many people tried to control one vision. Fullerton taught me how to continue performing when the room was not giving us much in return.

Donny taught me that another person's innovation did not threaten my experience. Johnny taught me that creative conflict could become growth if neither person walked away too quickly. Underneath all of it was recovery, although not in a loud or obvious way.

I was not standing onstage giving speeches about sobriety every night. I was learning how to live it through ordinary decisions. Could I listen when someone else had a better idea? Could I remain sober after heartbreak? Could I take a lower-paying job because the higher-paying one was damaging my spiritual health?

Could I admit that money had never saved me? Could I work beside people whose talents exposed my limitations? Could I stop treating every disagreement as a threat to my identity?

Sometimes I could, and sometimes I failed. The important thing was that I had begun asking the questions.

I still had plenty of ego, became resentful, wanted control, and remained emotionally immature in ways I did not completely understand. Sobriety had not turned me into a finished human being. It had given me the opportunity to grow.

By the end of that period, The Killer Dueling Pianos was still little more than a name. There was no major company, recognizable brand, national network of performers, patch, wine label, or large calendar filled with private and corporate events. There was no guarantee that any of it would ever happen.

What existed was a Facebook page, a few private shows, Donny, Johnny, and Steve waiting somewhere just beyond the edge of what I could see. More importantly, there was an idea I could not shake.

For most of my life, I had waited for someone else to give me the right opportunity. I had waited for a record deal, a better venue, a management position, a salary large enough to make me feel secure, or a relationship that would make me feel complete. None of those things had fixed me.

Maybe the next part of my life was not about finding the perfect place someone else had built. Maybe it was about building something myself.

At that point, I did not know how to do it. I only knew the name.

The Killer Dueling Pianos.

CHAPTER EIGHT

Build It Yourself

"Yes, I'm let loose, from the noose, that's kept me hanging around!"

SONG: BACK IN BLACK
BAND: AC/DC

The room in Fullerton was rarely full, but Johnny and I continued performing as though it were. Some nights there were enough people to create a little energy, and on other nights, the empty tables seemed to outnumber the customers. A packed room could carry an entertainer through a difficult night. A quiet room demanded that we generate everything ourselves.

Johnny and I were still learning how to work together. We had different instincts, different musical strengths, and different ideas about what made a dueling-piano show successful. I had been doing the work for years and carried strong opinions about how the format should be handled. Johnny had his own experience, an enormous catalog, and a stage presence that could not be ignored.

We did not always agree, but disagreement did not prevent us from improving. Johnny could play songs I did not know and approach familiar material in ways that would never have occurred to me. I could help shape the structure of the night and draw from everything I had learned during my years with Howl at the Moon. Over time, our differences became less of an obstacle and more of an advantage.

That was another lesson I had not learned easily. For most of my life, I had believed that the person in charge was supposed to have the best answer. If somebody else had a better idea, I felt exposed. Donny had already forced me to challenge that belief, and now Johnny was doing the same thing.

The room might have been small, but the education was significant. We learned how to hold people's attention when there were not many people to begin with. We learned how to adjust quickly, how to keep moving through a song that was not working, and how to create the feeling of a much larger show in a space that had very little energy of its own.

There is nowhere to hide when only a handful of customers are watching. In a large crowd, people sing over mistakes and help create momentum. In a quiet room, every pause feels longer, every weak choice becomes more obvious, and every performer has to work harder to establish a connection.

Johnny and I kept showing up. We slugged it out four nights a week and gave the people who came through the door the best show we could. At the time, it did not look like we were building anything important, but those nights developed the endurance we would need later.

The private events under The Killer Dueling Pianos' name continued arriving occasionally. They were not frequent enough to support me, and they certainly did not resemble a serious company. One event might come through a personal connection, followed by weeks or months when nothing happened.

Still, each private event taught me something. A bar show came with an established room, a staff, an audience that knew what it had walked into, and equipment that was usually already in place. A private event was different. The client expected us to arrive prepared, create the environment from nothing, and deliver an experience that justified whatever they had paid.

There was no permanent stage waiting for us. We had to think about instruments, sound, lighting, transportation, setup, timing, and communication with the client. If something was missing, we could not blame the venue or wait for another department to fix it. The responsibility followed us from the first phone call until the equipment was packed at the end of the night.

I did not yet have enough equipment to control the entire production myself. Sometimes we had to use whatever the venue provided, and sometimes we relied on rented or borrowed gear. That made every event unpredictable.

The name sounded larger than the operation behind it. The Killer Dueling Pianos suggested a complete entertainment company, but in those early years, the company was mostly me trying to put the right players in the right room with whatever resources were available.

I was still earning most of my income by working for someone else. The private events gave me a glimpse of independence, but they also showed me how unprepared I was to create it. Having a Facebook page and a company name did not mean I had a business.

I needed clients, equipment, performers, marketing, contracts, and a professional system. More than anything, I needed to stop waiting for somebody else to build those things for me.

Outside of music, I was becoming more connected to the motorcycle community. Riding had always given me a feeling of freedom that was difficult to explain to people who had never experienced it. On a motorcycle, the world did not disappear, but it became quieter. There was only the road, the machine, the weather, and whatever was directly in front of me.

I also found a sense of belonging among the people I met through riding. Rusty, Karina, and others in that community became part of my life. Loyalty mattered to them. Showing up mattered. A patch represented more than decoration because it connected the person wearing it to a larger group.

That idea stayed with me. Music companies did not normally think of themselves in those terms. Performers were often independent people who arrived for a show, collected their money, and moved on to the next opportunity. I began imagining something different, although I did not yet know exactly how to create it.

I wanted the people involved with The Killer Dueling Pianos to feel that they belonged to something. I did not want the company to be a random collection of musicians who happened to be available. I wanted it to have an identity, a standard, and a culture that people were proud to represent.

At that stage, however, the culture existed mostly in my head. I could imagine what the company might become, but imagination did not purchase equipment or create bookings.

By 2013, I had reached the point where I either had to make a serious investment or accept that The Killer Dueling Pianos would remain a side project. I decided to sell one of my motorcycles and put the money into the business.

Selling the motorcycle was difficult because riding meant more to me than transportation. It was part of my identity and one of the few things outside music that gave me a genuine sense of release. The decision forced me to choose between something I already loved and something I believed might become important.

I invested approximately ten thousand dollars into equipment. I bought piano shells, keyboards, a sound system, and the pieces we needed to walk into a private event without depending entirely on what the venue had available.

The piano shells mattered because appearance mattered. A pair of keyboards on stands could produce the music, but they did not create the visual impression people expected from a dueling-piano show. The shells allowed us to arrive looking like a complete production rather than a few musicians who had set up in the corner.

The sound system gave us greater control over what the audience heard. At a private event, poor sound could destroy the performance before the entertainers had a chance to connect with anyone. Owning the system meant I could not blame somebody else if it failed, but it also meant I could prepare it properly.

I developed a relationship with Casio as we expanded the equipment. Having reliable keyboards and a professional setup made it easier to present the company as something clients could trust. We were still small, but we no longer had to look small.

After buying the equipment, I had approximately twenty-eight hundred dollars left from the money I had set aside. I decided to spend it on Google advertising.

I did not fully understand Google advertising. I understood the basic promise: people searched for entertainment, our company appeared in front of them, and some of those people might become clients. What I did not understand was how quickly money could disappear when a campaign was not carefully managed.

I watched the balance drop at a speed that made me sick. Each click cost money, whether the person contacting us was serious or simply curious. I had taken money from the sale of my motorcycle, invested most of it in equipment, and was now watching the rest vanish into a system I barely understood.

My first reaction was panic. I thought I had made an expensive mistake and had nothing to show for it.

Then the phone began to ring.

Two national clients contacted me as a result of that advertising. Those inquiries did not instantly transform the business, but they showed me that people outside my existing network were searching for exactly what we offered. The problem had never been that there was no market. The problem was that the market did not know we existed.

That experience became another part of my education. I had spent most of my career believing talent created opportunity. Talent mattered, but people could not hire a company they had never heard of. A brilliant show hidden from the public was still a hidden show.

I had to learn how to market something, not simply how to perform it. That required a different set of skills, and most of them did not come naturally to me.

Onstage, I could read an audience and respond within seconds. In business, results often arrived slowly. I could make calls for days without receiving an answer, send messages that were ignored, and introduce the company to people who had no immediate interest.

Rejection onstage was temporary. One song could fail, and the next one might restore the room. Rejection in business could continue for weeks, with no applause or visible evidence that the work was leading anywhere.

My father helped me understand that part of it. He pointed out that the real value in sales was not simply receiving a yes. It was being willing to endure all the people who said no before the right person responded.

I began spending more time contacting venues, planners, clubs, and anyone else who might be able to use the show. I called it ground pounding because that was what it felt like. There was nothing glamorous about it. I was making calls, sending emails, introducing myself, following leads, and hearing no repeatedly.

Some people did not respond at all. Others seemed interested and then disappeared. A few wanted the entertainment but did not want to pay enough to support the performers and expenses involved.

I kept going because I understood that nobody was going to arrive and hand me a client list. If the company was going to grow, I would have to create those relationships one at a time.

During that same period, I needed hernia surgery. I had been assured that the Fullerton work would continue, which mattered because I was depending on the venue for regular income while the private business developed.

I scheduled the surgery believing I would have a position to return to once I recovered. Soon afterward, the venue closed its piano operation.

The timing was terrible. I was recovering physically, and the job I had expected to return to no longer existed. Earlier in my life, that combination could have become an excuse to collapse. I would have felt betrayed, blamed the people involved, and looked for something that would remove the fear.

I was angry and worried, but I stayed sober. More importantly, I began looking for the next workable opportunity instead of waiting for the old one to return.

The private company still could not fully support me, so I continued searching for regular venues. Work developed in and around Temecula, Murrieta, and Menifee. These were not massive rooms or prestigious national stages, but they gave us places to perform, develop the show, and introduce The Killer Dueling Pianos to new audiences.

Donny returned to the picture, and Johnny remained important. Steve Haas also became more involved. The people who would eventually form the center of the company were beginning to come together, although none of us could see the full shape of it yet.

Each performer brought something different. Donny had the voice, creativity, and instinct for entertaining that had impressed me from the beginning. Johnny had an enormous catalog and physical energy that could change a room. Steve had his own musical abilities and creative ideas.

My role was slowly changing. I was still a performer, but I was also becoming the person responsible for combining those different talents into a consistent experience.

That was more difficult than simply hiring good musicians. Talented performers did not automatically work well together, and a private client did not care how gifted each individual might be if the overall show felt disorganized. Somebody had to think beyond individual performances and protect the experience as a whole.

The years I had spent under other entertainment directors began making more sense. I had resented authority many times, but I was now discovering why structure mattered. A company needed expectations, communication, and standards. Without them, every performer would create a different version of the show, and the client would never know what they were purchasing.

At the same time, I did not want to recreate the environments that had made me miserable. I had worked for people who controlled every detail, dismissed new ideas, or expected loyalty without offering respect. I wanted standards without suffocating creativity.

Donny had already shown me how much the show could improve when I allowed another person to challenge the rules. Johnny had shown me that different musical instincts could strengthen a partnership. I needed to remember those lessons as I tried to lead.

That did not mean I always handled things well. I still became controlling when I was afraid, and fear was present constantly during those early years. Every event represented money I might not earn again. Every client felt important because I did not know when the next one would appear.

If a performer arrived late, changed something unexpectedly, or appeared unprepared, I did not experience it as a minor inconvenience. I experienced it as a threat to everything I was trying to build. Sometimes that fear came out as anger or rigidity.

Recovery required me to examine those reactions. I could not demand accountability from everyone else while refusing to examine my own behavior. I was responsible for the company, but responsibility did not give me permission to treat people badly.

My sponsor became an important voice during that period. I often complained about the companies I had worked for and the managers who, in my opinion, did not know what they were doing. I could describe every failure in detail and explain exactly how I believed the business should have been run.

Eventually, my sponsor challenged the pattern. If I believed I understood how performers should be treated and how an entertainment company should operate, then I needed to stop complaining and build one myself.

That did not mean I suddenly possessed all the knowledge necessary to do it. It meant I no longer had the right to hide behind criticism. Creating my own company would require me to test whether my ideas actually worked.

It is easy to judge somebody else's decisions when you are not carrying the consequences. Once I began carrying payroll, equipment costs, transportation, client expectations, and responsibility for the entire event, management looked different.

I still believed many of my former employers had made terrible decisions. The difference was that I could now understand how fear, financial pressure, and competing responsibilities influenced those decisions. Leadership was not simply choosing what seemed right in the moment. It was accepting the consequences after the choice had been made.

The venues in the Temecula area helped us develop a following. People who saw the show in a public setting began asking whether we could perform at weddings, fundraisers, corporate functions, and private parties. Every public performance became a form of marketing.

We began learning how different a private audience could be. In a piano bar, customers came because they already wanted entertainment. At a corporate event, some people were there because attendance was required. At a fundraiser, the entertainment had to support the larger purpose of the night rather than make itself the only focus.

Weddings created another set of expectations. The couple, families, planner, venue staff, and other vendors all had their own priorities. The show had to fit inside a larger event that could not be repeated if something went wrong.

Through the Temecula Valley wedding and events community, I met Annette Nielsen. She helped me understand aspects of the private-event business that I had not learned from years inside piano bars.

A private event began long before the first song. The client needed clear communication, realistic expectations, and confidence that we would arrive prepared. The venue needed information about space, power, timing, loading access, and sound requirements. Other vendors needed us to respect the schedule rather than behave as though the entire event revolved around our performance.

Contracts mattered. Timelines mattered. Presentation mattered. Returning calls mattered. The quality of the show was still essential, but professionalism began with everything that happened before we reached the stage.

That was not always comfortable for me. I enjoyed the creative work and the immediate response of an audience. Administrative details did not provide the same rush, but ignoring them could destroy the relationship with a client before we played a note.

I began building systems, although they were not sophisticated. I learned what information needed to be collected, what questions had to be asked, and what details could not be left until the day of the event.

Every mistake became part of the education. When something was forgotten, I tried to create a process that would prevent it from happening again. When a client misunderstood part of the agreement, I looked at how the communication could have been clearer.

I had spent years reacting to crises. Building the company required me to prevent some of them.

Country clubs became another market I believed could support the show. Their members wanted entertainment, many had established event calendars, and the venues were capable of hosting private functions.

I contacted country club after country club. Most of them did not respond, and many of the ones that did respond had no interest. I continued calling because one successful relationship could create repeat work and introduce us to people planning other events.

Calabasas Country Club became one of the early venues willing to give us an opportunity. That response validated months of outreach that had often felt pointless. The result did not come from one brilliant sales call. It came from continuing long enough to reach the person who was open to the idea.

That became the pattern of the company. People later saw the bookings, the travel, and the larger clients, but they did not see the unanswered messages that came before them. They did not hear the repeated no responses or watch me sit with the fear that I had invested money into a company nobody would hire.

Success usually looks cleaner when viewed from a distance. From inside it, the process was uncertain and frequently embarrassing.

I was learning new jobs every day. I was the entertainer, sales representative, equipment manager, scheduler, contract writer, and person clients called when something changed. I was also trying to remain active in recovery and maintain some form of personal life.

The company did not respect ordinary working hours. Clients called when they had time. Performers needed answers late at night. Equipment problems appeared during weekends, and venue questions often arrived while I was traveling to another show.

I answered because I was afraid not to. Every call might become a booking, and every booking might lead to another. The willingness to work helped the company grow, but it also revealed another part of my personality.

I could use work the same way I had used other things. It gave me somewhere to direct anxiety and allowed me to avoid questions I did not want to answer. As long as I was moving, calling, booking, performing, or repairing something, I did not have to sit still with myself for very long.

At the time, I mostly viewed that behavior as dedication. There was truth in that, but it was not the complete truth.

In 2015, I met a girl whom I'll call Red.

The relationship developed during a period when the company was still getting off the ground, but beginning to show real potential. My days were filled with building the business, but I still wanted the connection and security I had searched for throughout my life.

Red brought excitement and companionship. She became connected to the world I was creating, and I began imagining that the company and my personal life might grow together.

She wasn't sober when we met, but after a bad night, she began to pursue sobriety, which gave us an important point of connection. I understood how difficult early recovery could be and wanted to support her. Sharing that language created the feeling that we were moving in the same direction.

My own experience should have taught me that sobriety did not instantly create emotional maturity, but I still wanted to believe that shared recovery could protect a relationship from the problems I had experienced before. I saw the possibility of building something stable, both personally and professionally.

I was older than Red, much older, and the difference between our ages and life experiences was real. I had already lived through decades of addiction, professional collapse, and the early years of rebuilding. She was at a different stage of life.

Still, we became close. After years of traveling, temporary rooms, unstable relationships, and work that changed constantly, the idea of having someone beside me felt powerful.

The company was also expanding beyond what I could perform personally. A recurring opportunity in Lake Tahoe made that reality impossible to ignore.

For years, nearly every important show had depended on my presence. I believed I needed to be there to protect the quality, manage the client, and make sure the event represented the company properly. That approach might work for a performer, but it could never build a scalable business.

There were only so many nights I could perform and only one place I could be at a time. If every booking required me, the company would always remain limited by my calendar, health, and ability to travel.

The Lake Tahoe work forced me to trust other performers to carry the name without me. That was not easy. The company felt personal because it had grown from my experience, money, relationships, and years of rejection. Allowing another team to represent it felt like handing someone else a piece of my identity.

I worried that the performers might handle the show differently. I worried that a client might be disappointed because I was not present. I worried that one bad night could damage the reputation I had worked to establish.

Those fears were not completely irrational. A company's reputation could be affected by people the owner had trusted. The answer, however, could not be to control every show personally. The answer had to be choosing the right people, setting clear expectations, and allowing them to do what they did well.

Donny, Johnny, Steve, and the other performers were not copies of me. That was part of their value. Each of them brought something I could not provide, and the company became stronger when the show reflected those combined strengths.

The first times multiple teams performed in different locations felt strange. Somewhere, a client was watching The Killer Dueling Pianos without me in the room. The event carried the name I had created, used equipment connected to the company, and depended on performers I had trusted.

I could not step in if a song went wrong. I could not read the room for them, and I could not control every interaction with the client. All I could do was prepare the team and let them work.

When the events succeeded, my understanding of the company changed. It was no longer simply a name I used for my private shows. It was becoming something capable of existing without my physical presence.

That created an opportunity for everyone involved. Performers could work when I was booked elsewhere, clients could hire the company on more dates, and the business could accept opportunities that would otherwise have been impossible.

It also created new responsibilities. Scheduling became more complicated. Equipment had to be divided and transported. Different teams needed accurate information, and clients had to understand what they were purchasing.

I had to think beyond the show in front of me. One team might be performing in Lake Tahoe while another prepared for an event in Southern California. A problem in either place could still become my responsibility.

The pressure increased, but so did the possibility.

The website and promotional materials began taking on greater importance. A Facebook page had been enough when most bookings came from people who already knew me. A growing company needed a public presence that explained what we did and showed clients why our production was different.

Video was especially important because dueling pianos could be difficult to explain. People understood the words, but they did not always understand the energy, interaction, humor, or audience participation until they saw it.

We began creating material that showed the performance rather than simply describing it. The process was not perfect, and we were learning as we went. Still, every photograph, video, testimonial, and successful event gave the company more credibility.

The name began appearing in places where I had not personally introduced it. Clients referred us to other clients. Guests who saw the show at a private event contacted us for events of their own.

That was when the years of smaller rooms and unanswered calls began connecting. The public venues had taught us how to perform together. The early private events had taught us how to build a production. The failed advertising experiments had taught me that visibility mattered, and the repeated sales calls had created relationships that could lead to recurring work.

Nothing had happened as quickly as I wanted, but it was happening.

I also began understanding that the company could become a source of income for people I respected. Donny, Johnny, Steve, and the other performers were not simply helping me build my dream. They had their own responsibilities, families, and professional goals.

Every booking created work for somebody. That made each client more meaningful because the money no longer affected only me.

For much of my earlier career, I had measured success by what I received. The salary, title, applause, and attention were all evidence that I mattered. Building The Killer Dueling Pianos began changing that calculation.

Success could also mean creating an opportunity for somebody else. It could mean paying a performer properly, giving a client an experience they remembered, or building a relationship that produced work for years.

I was not always selfless about it. I still wanted recognition and worried constantly about money. I wanted the company to grow because its success made me feel secure and important.

Recovery had not erased those motives. It allowed me to recognize that more than one motive could exist at the same time. I could want success for myself while also becoming responsible for how that success affected others.

The company was still fragile. A few canceled events or equipment failures could create serious problems. I didn't have a large organization protecting me, and I was still learning most parts of the business through experience.

There were nights when the future seemed obvious and mornings when I wondered whether I had created something I could not sustain. Every new booking brought excitement, followed almost immediately by concern about how to execute it.

That cycle became normal. I learned to celebrate briefly and then return to the practical work required to fulfil the promise I had made to the client.

The business was growing because people enjoyed the performance, but it was surviving because we kept our commitments. Talent brought attention. Reliability created repeat clients.

That lesson connected directly to sobriety. My recovery had been built through repeated ordinary actions rather than one dramatic decision. I stayed sober one day at a time by continuing to do what had worked, even when I did not feel inspired.

The company developed in much the same way. There was no single event that transformed everything. We accumulated shows, relationships, equipment, experience, and trust.

Selling the motorcycle had not created a successful company by itself. The Google campaign had not created one. Calabasas Country Club, Lake Tahoe, and the Temecula venues had not created one individually either.

The company emerged from all of those decisions combined.

By the end of that period, The Killer Dueling Pianos no longer existed only in my imagination. We had equipment, promotional material, recurring clients, a growing group of performers, and the ability to operate more than one show.

Red was beside me, the company was expanding, and I had begun believing that I could create the kind of professional home I had never been able to find elsewhere.

For years, I had complained about other people's businesses. I had criticized their leadership, questioned their decisions, and imagined what I would do differently.

Now I had the opportunity to prove it.

That opportunity came with more fear and responsibility than I had expected, but it also gave me something I had spent my entire career searching for. I was no longer waiting for somebody else to decide whether I deserved a place on the stage.

We were building the stage ourselves.

CHAPTER NINE
The Patch

"So I've started out, for God knows where."

SONG: LEARNING TO FLY
BAND: TOM PETTY AND THE HEARTBREAKERS

By the end of 2015, The Killer Dueling Pianos was no longer just a name attached to whatever private work I could find. The company had a website, regular clients were beginning to call, and multiple performers were carrying the show into different rooms. For the first time, I could see evidence that the thing I had imagined might survive outside my own head.

The growth create d a new problem. We were becoming more visible, but we still did not look like a company with a clear identity. The dueling-piano industry had a familiar image, and most of it involved two men in ties or tuxedos sitting at polished pianos and delivering a clean, predictable version of the show.

That was not who I was, and it was not who the people around me were. We were musicians who had spent years in bars, bands, clubs, casinos, and every strange room that would pay us to play. We were loud, imperfect, tattooed, opinionated, and more interested in making a room explode than looking formal in a promotional photograph.

I wanted the company's image to reflect that.

At the time, the logo I had created was terrible. I had put something together using whatever basic design program I could manage, but there was nothing memorable about it. It served a temporary purpose, although it did not say anything about the company we were becoming.

Fortunately, Steve Haas was not only a talented musician. He was a real artist.

I asked Steve to create two designs. The first was a cleaner and more professional version of the basic company name. He produced something far better than anything I could have made on my own, but I also wanted another image that carried more attitude.

I had been around motorcycles and biker culture for much of my life. I understood the power of an image that could communicate identity before anyone said a word. A well-designed motorcycle patch did not look like a corporate logo. It looked like a statement.

I drew a rough idea on a napkin. Calling it a drawing is generous because it was barely more than a collection of lines showing Steve where I thought certain pieces might go. I told him to study biker patches and create something powerful, something that represented rock and roll, energy, and the attitude of the show.

People in the dueling-piano business had opinions about what would and would not appeal to clients. Some believed that brides and corporate planners wanted the safest possible image. According to that thinking, the entertainment had to appear polished, traditional, and harmless.

I did not want to build another company that looked exactly like everyone else's. I did not want people to see two older men in tuxedos and assume they already knew the entire show. I wanted them to see rock stars.

That did not mean the company would be unprofessional. The suits, contracts, timelines, and client expectations still mattered. The difference was that professionalism did not require pretending we were something we were not.

When Steve showed me the finished design, I could hardly believe what he had created from my terrible napkin sketch. The image had the edge and movement I wanted. It looked like music, motorcycles, and rock and roll had been forced into the same shape.

For the first time, I felt as though The Killer Dueling Pianos had a face.

The logo worked as marketing, but I wanted it to mean more than that. I had been burned by musicians before. I had worked with people who made commitments until something more attractive appeared, and I had watched performers treat a company as nothing more than another place to collect a check.

I did not want blind loyalty to me. I wanted commitment to the group.

The motorcycle world gave me a language for that idea. A patch could represent belonging, but belonging also created responsibility. It meant the person wearing it had agreed to support something larger than himself or herself.

That became the purpose of the Killer Dueling Pianos patch. A patched member was not simply someone I had hired for a show. It was someone who had made a commitment to the success of the company and to the other people carrying its name.

Steve was there for Johnny. Johnny was there for Donny. Donny was there for Steve. I was there for all of them, and they were there for me.

The patch did not mean we always agreed. It did not mean we never became angry, disappointed one another, or made mistakes. We were musicians, which guaranteed there would be strong personalities and occasional conflict.

It meant that conflict was not supposed to be the first excuse to disappear. It meant we handled the job, protected the client, and supported one another when life became difficult.

I was the only person in the company who regularly rode motorcycles, but the patch was never really about riding. It represented the brotherhood and sisterhood I had spent much of my life trying to find.

I had always felt slightly outside whatever group was considered normal. Even during the years when I was surrounded by people, I frequently felt alone. I could stand in front of a full room and receive applause while still wondering whether I truly belonged anywhere.

The company began giving me an answer. I was creating a place for musicians who were talented, independent, and sometimes as difficult to classify as I was.

Donny became central to that process.

Near the end of 2015, he told me he wanted to work more. I told him he could take the website and start selling the company, but sales did not interest him. What he wanted was better photography and better videos.

Up to that point, I had been doing much of the video editing myself. I knew enough to create something usable, but Donny saw what the material could become and approached it with the same intensity he brought to the stage.

I gave him room to do it, and he took over with a passion.

That was one of Donny's greatest qualities. Once he committed to something, he worked. He didn't need someone standing behind him reminding him to finish. He could spend hours sorting through performance footage, editing videos, and finding better ways to present the company.

Johnny and Steve were well suited to many of the local shows, while Donny gradually became my primary touring partner. We began spending more time on the road together, which meant we had to learn how to tolerate far more than one another's musical habits.

Donny and I are different in many ways. We don't vote the same. One of the jokes I bring up is that it's useless for either of us to vote, because our vote cancels the other's vote. He can barely finish a beer, while in my drinking days I could have finished all of mine and all of his without much difficulty.

None of those differences matter when the work begins. Donny is one of the hardest-working people I had ever met, and I trust his commitment.

He also understood the show in a way that went beyond playing songs. He knew that the audience needed movement, surprise, humor, and permission to participate. He could take a room that was holding back and pull it into the performance.

We still disagreed. There were creative decisions I would have handled differently, and I am sure there were days when he wondered why I had to make everything more complicated than it needed to be. The important part was that the disagreements did not stop the work.

By 2016, the company's calendar was expanding in several directions at once. The Lake Tahoe casino work continued, private weddings and corporate events increased, and fundraisers became a major part of what we did.

Some days, The Killer Dueling Pianos had three separate events happening at the same time. I might be traveling with Donny while Johnny and Steve handled another room and a different pair of performers carried the company somewhere else.

That level of activity would have been impossible only a few years earlier. At the beginning, I worried about finding one show. Now I had to think about how to cover several without lowering the quality of any of them.

The business also began stretching beyond California. A venue in Amarillo, Texas, wanted us to establish a regular show, and Donny and I started flying there approximately once every six weeks. Relationships developed in Texas and Oklahoma, creating more opportunities and expanding the group of musicians connected to the company.

Every new market introduced another set of problems. Equipment needed to be secured, local performers had to be evaluated, schedules had to be coordinated, and the client still expected the same experience regardless of how far the event was from my home.

The name had to mean something consistent.

That did not mean every performer had to become the same person. Donny, Johnny, Steve, and I had very different strengths, and forcing everyone into one style would have destroyed much of what made the company special.

Consistency meant that the energy, professionalism, and commitment were present even when the individual performers changed. The client needed to know that the people arriving under our name would show up prepared and take responsibility for the room.

That responsibility affected me differently now because the checks were no longer only for my own performances. I had players on payroll. People were receiving weekly income, and some of them were planning their schedules around work I had promised.

The company's success could help people, but my mistakes could also hurt them.

I thought about that constantly.

The revenue figures began reflecting how quickly things were changing. In 2013, the company had generated roughly thirty-six thousand dollars. The next year, that figure was around fifty-nine thousand, and by 2015, it had grown to approximately eighty-seven thousand.

Then the numbers jumped.

In 2016, company revenue increased to roughly two hundred and sixty-seven thousand dollars. By my recollection, 2017 came close to eight hundred thousand, 2018 was near nine hundred thousand, and 2019 reached approximately 1.1 million dollars.

Those figures represented company revenue, not money going directly into my pocket. Equipment, payroll, travel, insurance, advertising, taxes, and countless other expenses had to come out of it. Still, the growth was real, and it had happened faster than I ever expected.

It also meant there was never a natural point to stop.

Every new client suggested another possibility. One corporate event could lead to a convention, a fundraiser could introduce us to donors planning private parties, and a wedding guest could contact us months later about another celebration.

I answered every call because I was afraid the one I missed would become the opportunity that changed everything. I followed every lead because I remembered what it had felt like when nobody knew our name.

The company grew partly because I was willing to work when other people stopped. It also grew because I did not know how to stop working once there was something worth chasing.

During those building years, I did not take vacations. From 2016 through 2018, I was constantly traveling, performing, calling clients, handling schedules, solving problems, and making sure the next event was covered.

Some days lasted sixteen hours. On other days, I barely understood where one workday ended, and the next began. There was always another email, another contract, another performer who needed information, or another piece of equipment that had to reach a venue.

I told myself I was doing what every entrepreneur had to do. There was truth in that, but there was also another truth I did not want to examine too closely.

Work could numb me.

It did not affect my body in the same way alcohol or drugs had, but it gave me the same opportunity to avoid sitting still. As long as the company needed me, I did not have to spend much time thinking about whether I felt peaceful, secure, or emotionally whole.

I had learned how to build a life, but I was still learning how to live inside it.

The relationship with Red continued alongside the growth. She was patient with the hours I worked, especially considering how much of my attention went into the company. She also had needs and expectations of her own, and we frequently got on each other's nerves.

Our relationship was rocky at times. We broke up and got back together, argued about things that probably seemed small from the outside, and carried emotional differences that neither of us always knew how to discuss.

I believed I was going to marry her. I believed we would spend the rest of our lives together, and that belief affected nearly every personal decision I made.

The age difference between us remained real, as did the difference in our emotional development. I had more years behind me, but that did not automatically make me more mature. In relationships, some of the same insecurities I had carried since adolescence were still waiting for the right moment to take over.

Success did not fix them. Money did not fix them, and sobriety did not remove them simply because I had remained sober for several years.

Sobriety had given me the chance to recognize my behavior and take responsibility for it. It had not guaranteed that I would always respond well when I felt rejected, ignored, or afraid.

In 2016, I met Jamie McNeill, a dueling-piano performer based in Denver. Jamie had her own company and professional life, but we began working together and developed a close friendship.

She eventually became a patched member of The Killer Dueling Pianos. That distinction mattered to me because Jamie was not simply someone available for a booking. She became a sister to me and part of the group I trusted.

In 2018, Jamie and I performed at the Sturgis Motorcycle Rally in South Dakota. Combining music with the motorcycle world made that performance one of the highlights of my life.

I had spent years trying to build a company with an identity that felt natural to me. At Sturgis, the music, the patch, and the motorcycle culture came together in one place.

More important than the event itself was the friendship that continued developing between Jamie and me. She would become one of the people I knew I could call when life moved far beyond ordinary business problems.

That was what the patch was becoming.

It began as an image inspired by biker culture, but over time, it identified the people I considered family. We did not share parents, childhoods, or even the same home states, but we had shared stages, long drives, failed equipment, delayed flights, difficult clients, and the strange exhaustion that comes after giving everything to a room.

Those experiences created a bond outsiders did not always understand.

The business continued producing new branding opportunities. In 2018, we developed a relationship with Engelmann Cellars near Fresno. We had already been performing there, and that year the winery released a Zinfandel carrying The Killer Dueling Pianos label.

I had not had a drink in years, but I loved the marketing idea. Seeing the company logo on a wine bottle felt surreal. The image Steve had created was no longer only on our equipment or clothing. It had become something a client could hold, purchase, and remember.

The success should have made me feel completely satisfied.

From the outside, I had nearly everything I once believed would solve my problems. I had a growing company, money in the bank, performers who respected the work, and a woman I loved.

Inside, I was still capable of falling apart.

In 2018, Red wanted breast augmentation surgery. I paid approximately eight thousand dollars for the procedure. It was not necessarily the most emotionally mature decision I had ever made, but I wanted to make her happy.

Approximately six weeks later, she left.

I eventually learned that she had begun an online relationship with a man in England. By the time I understood what was happening, the emotional damage was already done.

I was furious about the other relationship, but underneath the anger was something much more basic. I wanted her back.

I didn't care about protecting my pride or proving that I could live without her. I did not want revenge, and I was not interested in hearing that I deserved someone better.

I wanted Red.

The company did not slow down because my relationship had ended. Contracts had already been signed, clients had dates on their calendars, and performers were depending on the work. Donny and I still had to get into vehicles, board planes, unload equipment, and walk onstage as though nothing had happened.

During the shows, I could function. Music still gave me a place to direct everything I was feeling, and the audience rarely knew what was happening after the last song.

Once the show ended, the pain returned.

Donny had to witness much of it. We spent so much time traveling together that there was nowhere for me to hide the emotional collapse. I cried, talked about Red, repeated the same thoughts, and became difficult to be around.

He remained steady when I was not.

I had never been in worse emotional shape up to that point. The company I had dreamed about was becoming successful, but I could not enjoy what I had built.

That was one of the cruelest parts of the experience. I could look at the growth and understand intellectually that something extraordinary was happening. I could see the bookings, revenue, performers, and recognition increasing.

Emotionally, none of it mattered because the person I wanted beside me was gone.

Earlier in my life, heartbreak would have led directly to drinking and drugs. I would have tried to erase the pain before I had a chance to understand it.

This time, I remained sober.

That statement can sound much more graceful than the experience actually was. Staying sober did not mean I accepted the breakup calmly or behaved like a spiritual master. I was angry, resentful, obsessive, and miserable.

I went to recovery meetings and talked to my sponsor. I continued praying and tried to follow the practices that had carried me through other periods of pain.

Most importantly, I asked God to place people in my life whom I could help.

I had learned in recovery that service could interrupt the endless cycle of thinking about myself. When I became trapped inside my own misery, helping another person gave me a reason to look outward.

I prayed for newcomers to appear. I asked God to put somebody in front of me who needed what had been given to me.

The prayer wasn't heroic. I was trying to survive myself.

Working with another person did not erase the heartbreak, but it gave the pain somewhere else to go for a while. I could talk to someone who was newly sober, listen to his fear, and remember that my life had once been much smaller than the problem currently consuming me.

Service reminded me that I still had something useful to offer, even when I did not feel useful.

There were days when I handled the loss better and days when I was extremely unpleasant to be around. I did not always carry the pain with dignity.

Recovery did not require me to pretend otherwise. It required honesty.

The honest truth was that I had built a company capable of making hundreds of people happy while feeling almost no happiness myself. I could bring energy into a ballroom, casino, winery, or fundraiser, then return to a hotel room and feel completely empty.

I began understanding that success and healing were not the same thing.

Success could change my finances, schedule, and professional reputation. It could create jobs and bring opportunities I had never imagined.

It could not do the emotional work for me.

Toward the end of 2018, after months apart, Red and I reconciled. I was so relieved to have her back that I did not care about analyzing everything that had happened.

I wanted to move forward.

At the house where I was renting a room, I arranged for us to have the larger master suite. The room gave us more space and felt like a small step toward building a life together again.

I was happy that she had returned, but the relationship remained rocky underneath that happiness. Reconciliation did not erase the insecurities or communication problems that had existed before she left.

I did not want to think about that. I wanted to believe that having her back was enough.

At the same time, the company was becoming more active in California's Central Valley. My first trip there had been in 2015, when a client named Mark Barlow hired us for his wife's birthday party.

At the time, Mark was only a client. He later became a friend.

I traveled north with a piano player named Liz, and the landscape affected me immediately. I had never spent much time in that part of California. The farms, open fields, and miles of carefully maintained almond trees felt completely different from the crowded parts of Southern California where I had been living and working.

There was peace in the Central Valley.

I remember wondering how I might eventually create a life in a place like that. At the time, moving there did not seem practical because I still depended heavily on Southern California venues and airports.

The thought remained.

We returned to the area for other events, including a fundraiser for the Visalia Elks Lodge. By 2018, one of the people connected to that event suggested that I consider purchasing a house in Visalia.

Brand-new homes were available there at prices that seemed impossible compared with Southern California. Red was also encouraging me to buy a house, although the idea made me nervous.

I had never owned one.

A house represented security, but it also represented commitment, maintenance, debt, and the possibility that I could lose what I had spent years building. In Southern California, the prices seemed irrational to me, and I did not want to commit myself to a mortgage simply because a bank said I could afford one.

I was approved for far more than I intended to spend. The lenders and real-estate people continued suggesting that I could buy a larger home, but their definition of affordability did not include the rest of my life.

They did not care whether I needed to eat, travel, maintain vehicles, care for pets, or keep the business operating. They saw the amount a bank was willing to lend.

I set my own limit at approximately two hundred and fifty thousand dollars.

There was one new house I particularly liked, but when I first saw it in November 2018, the asking price was approximately three hundred and five thousand dollars. I watched the price fall over the next several months, eventually reaching around two hundred and sixty-five thousand.

In January 2019, the builder held a red-tag sale, reducing the price to approximately two hundred and fifty-five thousand. Donny and I were in the area for a show and stopped to look.

It was raining, which kept many potential buyers away. Rain in California can make people act as though leaving the house is an unreasonable risk, but I was from Ohio and had no problem walking through it.

I told the sales office I wanted the house, but I also told them their price was still too high. I offered two hundred and forty thousand and wanted them to cover the closing costs.

They said the builder would never accept it.

I told them to submit the offer anyway. I had been laughed at before, and it no longer frightened me.

Donny and I left to continue our trip. Approximately fifteen minutes later, the phone rang, and I was told they would consider the deal if I used their lender.

That lender then stopped responding to me for nearly two weeks.

I had reached the point where I wanted the house, and being ignored made me furious. I called my own banking contact and asked him to handle it.

He negotiated the price to approximately two hundred and forty-five thousand, with the closing costs covered. From my perspective, the final cost came close to the number I had wanted in the first place.

My father had been encouraging me throughout the process. His advice was direct: "Buy the goddamn house."

In February 2019, I signed the papers on the first house I had ever owned. I put approximately fifty thousand dollars down because I wanted to reduce the additional requirements and keep the payment within a range that felt manageable.

I should have felt proud. Instead, Red became angry with me again shortly afterward and left for another period.

The house had been part of the life I imagined for both of us. Without her, it felt less like an achievement and more like an empty building I had committed myself to for decades.

I was still too busy to move in properly. The company had me performing four, five, and sometimes as many as six or seven shows in a week. I kept my place in the Temecula area because staying there was often cheaper than repeatedly paying for hotels when I had Southern California work.

Whenever I passed through Visalia, I stopped at the new house and walked through the empty rooms. There was almost no furniture, and nothing about the building felt like my life yet.

I wondered whether I could live there at all.

Part of the problem was that I had purchased it with Red in mind. I did not yet understand how to imagine a home that belonged to me alone.

Her parents later decided to move to Florida, and Red did not want to go with them. She told me she loved me and wanted to be with me.

In July 2019, she moved into the house and began working as a dog groomer in the Visalia area. I moved in more fully in September while continuing to keep the Temecula room for work.

We began decorating slowly. We bought furniture, explored Visalia, looked for places to eat, and found recovery meetings in the area.

We also argued about how the house should look. Those disagreements were rarely about furniture alone. Like many couples, we could turn small decisions into larger statements about who was being heard, who was in control, and whose version of the future mattered more.

I was paying for the house and the furniture, which affected how I viewed those arguments. Red was trying to make the place feel like her home too, which affected how she viewed them.

Neither perspective automatically made the other one disappear.

Even with those tensions, the house began to feel inhabited. We were no longer living out of one rented room while the company's equipment consumed the available space. There were separate rooms, a garage, and the possibility of building routines that were not based entirely on the next performance.

The neighborhood was still new. Only a few houses had been completed when I arrived, although more would eventually surround us.

I began meeting the people nearby, including Chris and Jenna and their three daughters on one side, and Scott and Samantha on the other. At the time, those were simply the neighbors I was getting to know.

I had no idea how important they would become.

Visalia also placed us close to the mountains. Sequoia and Kings Canyon National Parks were within reach, and Red sometimes went camping on her days off. When my schedule allowed, we traveled into the mountains together.

The peace I had noticed during my first Central Valley trip was still there. I simply did not have much time to experience it.

The company was moving faster than ever.

By 2019, we were performing approximately two hundred shows a year. By my count, I had around thirty-nine piano players connected to the company across the country and receiving payroll.

There were more opportunities than I could fill. I had spent years begging venues to return my calls, and now I had to turn work down because there were not enough qualified performers available on certain dates.

That created a different kind of anxiety. Saying no to a client still felt dangerous because I remembered how quickly work could disappear. I wanted to accept every opportunity, but accepting a show without the right team would have damaged the reputation that had created the opportunity in the first place.

The calendar for 2020 was already filling. Based on the work coming in, I believed company revenue might reach somewhere between 1.5 and two million dollars.

It felt like the years of risk, rejection, and exhaustion were finally producing the life I had imagined.

At home, I wanted to celebrate Christmas.

I had not truly celebrated it in more than a decade. I had seen family at times and participated in parts of the holiday, but I had not created a Christmas in a home of my own.

Now I had a place where I could put up a tree.

That desire may sound simple, but it carried more emotional weight than I understood. The house represented permanence, something I had rarely experienced. A Christmas tree meant I was no longer passing through somebody else's room, hotel, or temporary arrangement.

It meant I lived there.

Red and I celebrated Christmas in the new house in December 2019. For a while, it felt as though the different parts of my life were finally occupying the same space.

The business was successful. Red was with me. I owned a home, had money in the bank, and could imagine a future that did not involve losing everything I touched.

On December 26, we brought home a black cat and named her Sophie Olivia Christmas. In January, we brought home another cat, Meg, whom we named Megan Elizabeth New Year.

I had grown up with cats, but I was not completely sure about bringing animals into the new house. I traveled constantly, and I understood the additional responsibility.

We did it anyway.

The cats began changing the house almost immediately. A building can be clean, furnished, and expensive without feeling alive. Animals do not care what the mortgage costs or whether the furniture matches. They simply begin treating the place as home.

By the beginning of 2020, the company calendar was stacked with work. Red and I had a house, the cats were settling in, and the patch I had once imagined as a symbol had become part of a national group of performers.

Everything looked secure.

I had spent years trying to create something no employer, relationship, or bad decision could take from me. The business had survived my inexperience, financial fear, surgeries, venue closures, and heartbreak. It had grown because we had kept working when there was no evidence the work would pay off.

I believed we had finally reached the point where momentum would carry us forward.

The dates were booked. The contracts were signed. Performers across the country were depending on the calendar, and I was preparing for the largest year the company had ever experienced.

For once, the future did not look uncertain.

It looked full.

CHAPTER TEN

The Day the Music Stopped

"Tried to fly, but we climbed too high."

SONG: ALL FOR YOU
BAND: MOTORHEAD

On March 13, 2020, Donny and I performed at a fundraiser in the Central Valley for a woman participating in the Leukemia & Lymphoma Society's Woman of the Year campaign. Her family had hired us before, and the event was the kind of work The Killer Dueling Pianos had spent years building toward. It brought together entertainment, community, and fundraising, three things that had become central to the company.

The show itself did not feel like the end of anything. We arrived, set up, performed, and helped raise money. The woman we were supporting would eventually win her campaign, although nobody knew that at the time. For us, it was another successful event on a calendar already filled with work.

By then, the news had been full of reports about a new virus spreading through the country. Events were beginning to change; people were canceling travel, and there was talk about closing businesses for a short period. The language being used suggested that the shutdown might last two weeks.

I did not believe two weeks would solve anything, but I also did not understand what was coming. Nobody did.

As I drove home across the Central Valley after the fundraiser, the atmosphere felt different. The roads were familiar, but there was an uncertainty underneath everything. News reports were changing by the hour, and people were beginning to empty stores as though normal life might disappear overnight.

At approximately one in the morning, I stopped at a twenty-four-hour Walmart. The shelves had already been picked through, so I bought whatever food remained that Red and I might be able to use. The people at the fundraiser had also sent me home with a couple of racks of beef, which suddenly felt much more valuable than leftovers from an event.

I drove home with groceries and meat in the vehicle, still trying to understand what the next few weeks might look like. I had spent years building a business around rooms filled with people, and now people were being told to stay away from one another.

At first, Red and I tried to treat the shutdown as a temporary interruption. I had been traveling constantly for years, sometimes performing five or more shows in a week. We told ourselves that having me home for a short period might even be good for us.

Red was still working as an animal groomer. Where we lived, animal care was treated as necessary work, so she continued going into the grooming salon while my industry stopped almost immediately.

I suddenly had more time at home than I had experienced in years. I could ride my motorcycle, spend time with Sophie and Meg, and finally live inside the house I had purchased more than a year earlier. Until then, I had been home only two or three nights during many weeks.

Part of me was still trying to enjoy the fact that the house was new. I had walked through those rooms when they were empty, wondering whether I would ever truly live there. Even after moving in, I had been traveling so often that the place sometimes felt more like a property I owned than a home I inhabited.

I wanted to enjoy the new paint smell. I wanted to sit in the house without checking the clock to see when I had to leave for another airport, venue, or long drive.

There were moments during those first weeks when Red and I managed to make the best of it. We ordered food, and I sometimes went out to bring sushi home. We watched the daily updates and tried to understand which warnings were serious and which information would change by the next morning.

When Red returned from work, I worried about what she might bring inside from the salon. I would meet her at the door, have her remove her work clothes, and put everything directly into the washing machine. At the time, we did not know how the virus spread or how much danger was attached to every surface.

Fear made ordinary actions feel dangerous. A grocery bag, a package, a pair of work clothes, or a trip outside could become something to analyze.

I tried to remain positive because I was responsible for more than myself. The Killer Dueling Pianos had performers across the country, and many of them depended on the company for income. They had bills, families, rent, and groceries to purchase, just as I did.

On the night of that final fundraiser, I sent one hundred dollars to every performer on my payroll. By my recollection, there were roughly thirty-two people at the time. The amount was not enough to solve anyone's problems, but it might help them buy groceries while we waited to see what happened.

I told them to get some food. None of us knew how long we were going to be unable to work, and I still believed there was a possibility that the calendar would restart after a short pause.

It did not restart.

The cancellations began almost immediately. One client called, followed by another, and then the emails began arriving. Weddings, fundraisers, corporate events, conventions, private parties, and recurring venue shows were all being canceled or postponed without any reliable future date.

In contract language, the situation fell under force majeure. These were circumstances outside anyone's control. The clients had not created the pandemic, and neither had I. Many of them were frightened about their own businesses, jobs, and families.

They still wanted their deposits returned.

Each deposit represented an event I had already planned around. Performers had been assigned, equipment had been arranged, travel had been considered, and the date had been removed from our availability. The money in the company's accounts was connected to work we had expected to complete.

Now the work could not happen.

One by one, I returned the deposits. By the time the cancellations slowed, I had refunded over $130,000 from the company's accounts.

Watching that money leave was terrifying. The financial growth of the previous years had given me some protection, and I was not broke, but there was an enormous difference between having money and watching an entire source of income disappear.

The company's income fell by approximately ninety-five per cent. We went from performing around five shows a week to having almost nothing.

Every phone call became something I dreaded. Before the pandemic, an unknown number might have represented a new client. Now it was usually somebody asking whether an event was still happening or requesting money back.

Performers also called wanting to know whether their shows were going forward. I hated giving them the answer because I understood what the cancellation meant to them.

"No, that gig's not fucking happening," I had to tell them, sometimes repeatedly during the same day.

There was nothing I could offer in its place. I could not move the show to another venue because every venue was facing the same problem. I could not promise another date because nobody knew when events would return.

The collapse was made more stressful by changes I had already been forced to make inside the company. New California employment rules had taken effect at the beginning of 2020, requiring me to restructure the way performers working in the state were classified and paid.

Getting the company compliant had cost me close to $25,000. I had spent the money believing 2020 would be our largest year and that the number of bookings would cover the additional expense.

Instead, I entered the shutdown after paying tens of thousands of dollars to restructure the business, only to discover that there might no longer be a functioning business to restructure.

For years, I had complained that I could never stop working. Now I discovered that being forced to stop was much worse.

The company had become the structure around nearly every part of my life. It determined where I traveled, who I spoke to, how I earned money, and what I did when I woke up each morning. The constant calls and problems exhausted me, but they also gave me a sense of purpose.

When the work disappeared, the purpose became harder to find.

There were no hotels to book, no sound checks, and no stages waiting for us. Equipment sat unused while the contracts connected to it vanished. The performers I had worked so hard to bring together were scattered across the country with no idea when they might see one another again.

The patch had represented commitment. I had told people that we were a brotherhood and sisterhood and that we would be there for one another. Now I was confronting a situation where loyalty alone could not produce work.

I could send a little money and answer their calls, but I could not reopen the country. I could not force clients to hold events, and I could not protect everyone from what was happening.

That helplessness was difficult for me. I had built my entire adult identity around solving problems. If equipment failed, I replaced it. If a performer canceled, I found another player. If a client needed something, I figured out how to provide it.

This problem didn't care how hard I worked.

It didn't respond to another phone call, another advertisement, or another sixteen-hour day. There was no person I could persuade and no room I could walk into and win over.

For the first time since starting the company, effort and results had been completely disconnected.

I spent more time following the news than was healthy for me. Every announcement seemed to produce another rule, another cancellation, or another reason the entertainment industry would remain closed.

I became angry at the people making those decisions. From my perspective, the damage being done to small businesses, musicians, people in recovery, and others living on the edge of emotional survival was not being treated as seriously as it should have been.

I understood that people were frightened of the virus, especially during the early weeks when nobody seemed to know exactly what we were dealing with.

What made me furious was the feeling that the people ordering businesses to close didn't have to live with the consequences in the same way we did. My accounts were being drained by refunds, my employees had lost their work, and the company I had sacrificed years to build had been reduced to a calendar of canceled dates.

My anger didn't improve anything. It gave me somewhere to direct the fear, but it didn't reopen a single venue.

At home, the pressure was beginning to change the relationship between Red and me. I had initially believed that spending more time together might help us reconnect. Instead, the absence of work removed the distance that had sometimes allowed us to avoid unresolved problems.

Before the shutdown, I was gone five days a week, much of the time. Red had lived in the house more consistently than I had since moving there in July 2019. She had developed her own routines while I traveled, and now I was suddenly present every day.

I wanted to experience the house as something new. She had already been living in it for months.

That difference sounds small, but many of our arguments began with small things. The way a room was arranged, how something was cleaned, where an item belonged, or what needed to be done around the house could become connected to much larger resentments.

I was paying for the house, furniture, and most of the expenses. The business that made those payments possible had almost completely stopped producing income. I felt the pressure of protecting everything financially, and I did not believe Red fully understood how much responsibility I was carrying.

From her perspective, I had suddenly become a constant presence inside a space where she had built a daily life. I was anxious, angry, and watching money leave the company every day. I was not easy to live with.

There were still good moments between us, but the tension became harder to ignore. Red's parents were living in Florida, and she spoke with her mother frequently through FaceTime. From what she saw and heard, life there appeared less restrictive than it felt in California.

She didn't have a large circle of close friends in Visalia. The shutdown made that isolation worse, and the person she was around most of the time was me.

I loved her deeply, but love did not prevent resentment from growing. We had many things in common and had spent five years trying to make the relationship work. We had also developed patterns that neither of us knew how to interrupt.

I became frustrated about money, responsibility, and the future. Red had her own frustrations, and instead of discussing them in a way that brought us closer, we often allowed them to turn into arguments.

Our physical relationship began fading as well. Resentment and intimacy do not coexist easily. It is difficult to feel close to someone while silently keeping track of everything you believe that person does not understand about your life.

The lack of physical connection created another form of rejection between us. I didn't always recognize how Red was experiencing it, and she could not automatically understand everything happening inside me.

Neither of us was handling the situation well.

The pandemic had taken away nearly every outlet I normally used to manage stress. I could not perform regularly, travel, stand in front of an audience, or disappear into the work of the company.

I remained sober, but I was discovering that sobriety did not guarantee emotional balance. The behaviors I had used to avoid difficult feelings had changed over the years, but the need to escape them was still present.

Work had become one of those forms of escape. When I was traveling, I could postpone a difficult conversation because I had a plane to catch or a show to perform. When I returned home exhausted, I could tell myself there was no time to deal with relationship problems.

Now there was nothing but time.

The silence inside the house made every unresolved issue louder.

For most of April, I continued expecting an announcement that would allow events to resume. Every day felt like it might be the day someone finally provided a clear plan.

Instead, the dates continued moving. Two weeks became a month, and a month began stretching into an unknown period.

At the end of April, local officials where I lived indicated that they were not interested in aggressively closing every business. The Central Valley did not respond to the restrictions in the same way as some of California's larger cities.

That gave us a little hope.

Engelmann Cellars in Fresno was one of our favorite venues. The owners had supported the company for years, hosted our shows, and worked with us on The Killer Dueling Pianos wine label.

We had an outdoor performance scheduled there for May 30. Rather than canceling, the venue decided to move forward with the event while spreading people across the outdoor area.

Approximately six hundred people attended.

Walking onto a stage again felt like returning to the part of myself that had been missing. For a few hours, there was music, an audience, and the familiar exchange of energy between the performers and the people watching.

The crowd was spread out, but they were there. They wanted entertainment, and we wanted to give it to them.

I had spent years learning that music could provide relief during difficult moments. I had seen it after September 11 and during fundraisers for people facing illness or loss. People sometimes needed permission to laugh, sing, and forget what frightened them for a while.

That show reminded me why the company mattered.

It did not, however, mean the business had returned. Before the pandemic, I might have performed five times during an ordinary week. During the summer of 2020, the company was sometimes working only two or three times in an entire month.

The May performance was an exception, not a reopening.

When the equipment was packed and the crowd went home, the calendar remained nearly empty. I returned to the house and the same financial and relationship pressures that had been waiting before the show.

The contrast was difficult. Onstage, I could briefly feel like the person I had been before March. At home, I was still watching the life I had built come apart.

Early in June, Red and I went into the mountains together. We had a good day, and for a little while, it felt possible that we might find our way back to each other.

The Central Valley had been one of the things that initially attracted me to the area. The fields and mountains carried a sense of peace that Southern California rarely gave me. I had imagined that buying the house near those places would help us build a quieter life.

A few days after the mountain trip, Red and I argued again.

The subject of the argument mattered less than what had accumulated beneath it. Months of financial fear, isolation, resentment, and physical distance were sitting behind whatever words we exchanged.

Red called her mother and said she was going to Florida.

At first, I understood that her transfer might take a few weeks or perhaps a month. That gave me time to believe I could change her mind.

I begged her not to go. I pleaded, cried, and tried to explain how much I loved her. After everything we had survived together, I could not accept that the relationship might end during the same period when the company was collapsing.

The fear of losing her was not new. I had experienced it when she left in 2018 and during the other unstable periods in our relationship. When she returned, I had convinced myself that we had survived the worst of it.

Now the fear was back, and it was happening inside the house I had bought for the future I imagined we would share.

I wanted to do something that would show Red I was still committed to that future. I had money, despite the losses the company was experiencing, and I decided to put a swimming pool in the backyard.

The decision was not completely rational. I was frightened, desperate, and trying to create a reason for her to see a life with me in that house. The pool represented summers, family, friends, and a home that could become more than a building where two unhappy people argued.

I signed a contract to have it built. The project would cost approximately fifty thousand dollars.

I believed I was investing in us. In reality, I was attempting to solve an emotional crisis with another major financial commitment.

Around the middle of June, Red came home from work and told me the transfer had been approved much faster than expected. She would be leaving that Sunday.

There was no longer a month in which I could persuade her to reconsider. There were only a few days.

She began packing everything she could fit into her car. I watched five years of our life being reduced to whatever she could take with her.

I cried and begged her to stay. I reminded her of everything we had built and everything we had planned. None of it changed her decision.

Red wanted to take Sophie with her. Sophie had initially been more closely attached to me, while Meg had developed a strong connection with Red. The cats, however, were bonded to each other.

They groomed one another, slept beside each other, and had never known life apart. I could not accept the idea of separating them or sending one of them across the country during a hot and unstable summer.

I told Red she could not take Sophie. The cats were legally in my name, and I believed keeping them together was the right decision.

That moment added another painful layer to the departure. Red was leaving without the relationship, the house, or either of the animals she had helped bring into it.

I understood that she was hurting too. At the time, however, I could barely see beyond my own panic.

When the day arrived, she packed the car and left for Florida.

After five years of trying to make the relationship work, it ended without the kind of conversation that provides closure. There was no mutual acceptance that we had reached the end, and there was no promise that we would remain friends.

She drove away while I remained in the house.

The next day, Red sent me a message. She told me that she was driving through towns I had called her from during years of traveling for shows.

I imagined those places differently when she mentioned them. They had once represented the work I was doing to build our future. I had called her from hotel rooms, venues, highways, and cities across the country because I wanted her to remain connected to my life while I was away.

Now she was moving through those same places in the opposite direction, leaving that life behind.

I begged her again to come home.

She did not.

After that, I never heard from her again.

For five years, Red had been part of nearly every plan I made. Even when the relationship was unstable, I had continued imagining that the two of us would eventually find a way to make it work.

I had not prepared for a future in which she disappeared completely.

The house changed the moment she left. The rooms were the same, but everything inside them seemed connected to her. Furniture we had chosen, spaces we had argued over, and ordinary household items all became reminders that she was gone.

Meg understood that something had changed, even if she could not understand why. For 3 days, she walked through the house meowing loudly and searching the rooms for Red.

Watching her was unbearable.

I could not explain to an animal that the person she was looking for had driven across the country and was not coming back. Every time Meg entered another room and cried, I broke down again.

I had spent most of my life believing animals were resilient because they could not describe their feelings in words. Watching Meg search the house showed me how wrong that assumption was.

She knew someone was missing.

Sophie and Meg became one of the reasons I did not immediately sell the house. I wanted out of it. I did not care whether I lost money because the property no longer represented security.

It represented failure.

I had purchased it for a life with Red, and now I was living inside the evidence that the life had not worked. The mortgage, furniture, and rooms all felt connected to a decision I could no longer undo.

Selling the house would have created another disruption for the cats. They had only recently begun treating it as their permanent environment, and I could not bear the thought of separating or rehoming them.

They had lost Red. I did not want them to lose each other and the only home they knew.

Outside, workers began digging the pool.

The contract had already been signed, and the project continued even though the future it was meant to serve no longer existed. Every stage of the construction reminded me that I had committed approximately fifty thousand dollars to an attempt to save a relationship that had ended before the first person entered the water.

I resented the machinery, the hole in the yard, and the money leaving my account. The pool was supposed to make the house feel complete, but as it took shape, the house felt emptier than ever.

I stopped sleeping in the bedroom. The room carried too much of the relationship, and being inside it made the loss impossible to escape.

I slept on the couch instead.

The business remained nearly silent. There were no full weeks of performances to pull me away from the house, and there was no audience waiting to distract me from what had happened.

For years, I had survived heartbreak by continuing to work. This time, the heartbreak and the disappearance of work had arrived together.

I stayed sober. Drinking was not going to bring Red back, reopen the venues, restore the calendar, or stop Meg from searching the rooms.

Knowing that did not make sobriety feel comforting. It only meant I had to experience everything without the escape I once would have used.

I talked about the breakup with anyone willing to listen. I wrote, called people in recovery, and attempted to understand what had happened. I examined my behavior and knew I had made mistakes.

I had allowed financial pressure to become resentment. I had not always communicated with kindness, and I had responded to rejection and fear in ways that pushed us further apart.

Accepting my part did not mean I believed every part of the ending was my fault. It meant I could not survive by making Red responsible for everything I felt.

That understanding came slowly. During those first days, I was simply broken.

By the middle of 2020, nearly every part of the life I had celebrated six months earlier had changed. The calendar that had once looked full was empty, the performers connected to the company had almost no work, and the woman I believed I would marry had left the state.

The house was still standing, but it did not feel like home. The company still legally existed, but there was almost no music.

Outside, a swimming pool was being built for a future that had disappeared before the construction began. Inside, Meg continued looking for Red, Sophie stayed beside her, and I slept on the couch because I could not bring myself to enter the bedroom.

At the end of 2019, I had believed momentum would carry us forward. By the summer of 2020, the stages were dark, the house was quiet, and all I could hear was the machinery digging a hole in the backyard.

CHAPTER ELEVEN

The Black Heart

"Ooh, a storm is threatening, my very life today."

SONG: GIMME SHELTER
BAND: THE ROLLING STONES

After Red left, I remained in the house because of Sophie and Meg. I had wanted to sell it immediately, even if that meant losing money, because every room reminded me of the future I had imagined with her. The cats had already lost one of the people who had raised them, however, and I could not make them lose their home too.

They were inseparable. They groomed each other, slept together, followed each other through the rooms, and seemed to understand when the other one was distressed. I had watched Meg search for Red for days, crying as she moved through the house, and I did not want either cat to experience another separation.

Protecting them gave me a reason to stay, but it did not make the house feel like mine. I continued sleeping on the couch because I could not bring myself to sleep in the bedroom. I had purchased the house while imagining a life with Red, and the bedroom held too many reminders of that life. It felt easier to remain in the living room, where I could hear the cats moving nearby and pretend I was only there temporarily.

Outside, workers continued building the swimming pool I had ordered while trying to save the relationship. The contract had already been signed, the money had already been committed, and the construction was moving forward even though the purpose I had attached to it was gone.

Every time I looked into the backyard, I saw a large hole representing approximately fifty thousand dollars and one of the most desperate decisions I had ever made. I had imagined Red and me sitting beside that pool, entertaining friends, and creating a life in the house. Instead, I watched strangers dig it while she drove farther away.

The company remained nearly silent. There were occasional shows, but nothing close to the schedule we had maintained before the pandemic. I had spent years complaining that I was too busy, only to discover how much of my identity depended upon being needed.

When the phone stopped ringing with new bookings, I did not know what to do with myself. There were still calls from clients trying to move dates, performers asking when work might return, and people wanting to know what I believed would happen next. I had no answers for them because I did not have any answers for myself.

For most of my adult life, music had provided structure. Even during the worst periods of addiction, there had usually been a stage waiting somewhere. Recovery had later given me meetings, commitments, prayer, and service. Building the company added an endless schedule of calls, travel, contracts, equipment, and performances.

Now the stages were dark, the recovery meetings had moved online, and the woman I loved had disappeared from my life. The structures that had held me upright were either gone or had become distant versions of themselves.

I stayed sober, but sobriety did not make me feel grateful to be alive.

I was not planning to kill myself. I understood the devastation suicide left behind because I had seen what it did to families and friends. I could not deliberately place that pain onto my parents, brothers, nieces, friends, neighbors, performers, or the people in recovery who depended upon me. I also could not imagine what would happen to Sophie and Meg if I were gone.

Even so, I no longer saw much value in my own life. There is a difference between deciding to end your life and wishing you would not wake up, although the darkness behind those thoughts can come from the same place.

After Jenn died, I had begun including her in my nightly prayers. I still prayed to God on my knees beside the bed, as I had since getting sober, but I also spoke to Jenn. She had become part of my spiritual life, someone I carried with me even though she was no longer physically present.

During those months after Red left, my prayers changed. I began asking God to take me in my sleep.

I didn't want to hurt myself. I wanted God to make the decision for me. I wanted to go to sleep and be released from the anger, heartbreak, isolation, and sense that everything meaningful had been taken away at once.

Some nights I prayed to Jen too. I had spent years talking to her, asking for guidance and remembering the grace she showed while dying. During the pandemic, I asked why I was still here when I no longer understood what I was supposed to be doing.

My heart felt black. That was the only way I knew how to describe it.

It didn't feel temporarily bruised or merely broken. It felt as though something inside me had closed and hardened. I didn't want encouragement, slogans, or reminders that other people had things worse. I already knew I had a house, money, family, friends, and two cats who loved me. I understood that many people had lost far more than I had.

Gratitude could not reach the place I was in.

People sometimes use gratitude as though it should cancel every other emotion. They believe that if you can identify enough good things in your life, you will lose the right to feel despair. That was not how it worked for me. I could recognize everything I still had and remain incapable of feeling connected to it.

My anger became almost as consuming as the heartbreak. I blamed the people making decisions during the pandemic for destroying businesses, isolating people in recovery, and removing the connections that had kept many of us stable. I watched people I knew fall back into addiction, and I heard about sober people taking their own lives.

Every new shutdown announcement intensified that rage. I believed that the people ordering restrictions didn't understand what prolonged isolation was doing to musicians, business owners, recovering addicts, and people already struggling with depression.

Whether my anger was helping anybody did not matter to me at the time; it gave me somewhere to place the pain, and I had an enormous amount of pain requiring somewhere to go.

The more I followed the news, the angrier I became. The angrier I became, the more isolated I felt. I could spend hours thinking about everything being done to us and then lie awake on the couch, unable to change any of it.

Recovery had taught me that resentment was dangerous, but knowing that didn't automatically remove it. I had used the tools of recovery long enough to understand what I was supposed to do. I could write about the resentment, examine my part, pray for the people I hated, call my sponsor, and try to be of service.

I did some of those things, but I didn't always do them willingly. There were nights when I had no interest in forgiveness because anger felt like the only remaining proof that I cared about what had happened.

The recovery meetings moving online made everything more difficult. I continued attending, but the connection did not feel the same through a screen. People appeared as small boxes, sometimes with their cameras turned off, and the informal conversations that happened before and after meetings nearly disappeared.

A recovery meeting had never been only about the formal discussion. It was also the person who noticed you seemed different, the hand on your shoulder, the conversation in the parking lot, and the newcomer who stayed behind because he was afraid to go home alone.

Online meetings preserved part of the structure, but they could not recreate all of that human contact. The quality of my connection to the recovery community declined at the exact time I needed that connection most.

Unexpectedly, the people living around me began filling some of the space.

When I bought the house, the neighborhood was still developing. Chris and Jenna lived on one side with their three daughters. Scott and Samantha lived on the other side, while Casey and Lauren lived near the corner of the cul-de-sac. At first, they had simply been the people whose houses happened to surround mine.

I had lived in California long enough to know that proximity did not always create a relationship. People could share a wall, driveway, or property line for years and know almost nothing about one another. Everyone entered a garage, closed the door, and returned to a private world.

Our street became different.

With travel reduced and everyone spending more time close to home, we began talking more. Short conversations outside grew into actual relationships. The people I had known as neighbors gradually became the people checking whether I was all right.

Chris and Jenna became especially important. Chris was intelligent, practical, and someone I could speak to about subjects far beyond the ordinary conversation between neighbors. Jenna and their daughters brought warmth into a period when the house beside them held very little.

They could not replace my family, and I was not estranged from my parents or brothers. My family remained supportive, but they lived far away. There is a difference between somebody loving you from another state and somebody being able to walk across the yard when you are falling apart.

My neighbors were physically present. They saw me on the days when I could not disguise what I was feeling, and they continued treating me like a person worth caring about.

I didn't always understand why.

I could perform for a room full of strangers without difficulty, but receiving quiet care from people nearby made me uncomfortable. There was no applause attached to it and nothing I had done to earn it. They were simply showing up because they had decided I mattered to them.

The cats helped create connections too. Sophie and Meg became known around the neighborhood, and the people close to me understood how important they had become. When I eventually began traveling again, Chris, Jenna, and their daughters would help care for them.

At that moment, however, I was rarely going anywhere. Most days it was just the three of us inside the house.

Sophie and Meg developed their own routines around me. They followed me, slept close by, and seemed to notice when I was distressed. I had kept the house partly to protect them, but the truth was that they were protecting me too.

Caring for animals required me to perform small acts of responsibility even when I did not care what happened to me. They needed food, clean water, litter boxes, attention, and stability. I could wish not to wake up while still making sure everything was ready for them before I went to sleep.

Those ordinary responsibilities kept me connected to life in ways I didn't fully appreciate at the time.

Around that period, my niece Maddie came to visit. I cannot remember with certainty whether the visit happened late in 2020 or sometime in 2021, but I remember what her presence felt like. Maddie was a bright light, and having her in the house interrupted the isolation for a while.

Family members often don't realize how much a simple visit can matter to somebody who has been alone for too long. She didn't need to solve anything. Her presence reminded me that there were relationships in my life not defined by business, recovery, or romantic failure.

The brightness of the visit did not last after she left. I returned to the same house, the same couch, and the same prayers at night.

Christmas arrived in 2020, and I wanted nothing to do with it. The previous Christmas had been the first real holiday I had celebrated in my own home. Red and I had decorated, brought Sophie home the day after Christmas, and added Meg to the family shortly after New Year's.

One year later, Red was gone, the company was barely operating, and the house felt like a monument to everything that had collapsed. I didn't decorate or try to recreate what we had done the year before.

My family pushed me to join a FaceTime call for Christmas. I didn't want to participate, and once I joined, I could not pretend to be cheerful. I was not interested in performing happiness for the people who loved me.

They wanted to see me, but I wanted the day to end. I had spent most of my professional life creating celebrations for other people. That Christmas, I could not create one for myself.

The thoughts about death continued, but another thought had begun appearing alongside them. Before Red left, I had occasionally imagined myself seriously ill and in a hospital. I didn't know what the illness was, and I had no medical reason to believe anything was wrong.

The images disturbed me partly because I had always handled the practical details in the relationship. I paid the bills, ran the company, and managed the problems. I wondered how Red would respond if I became terminally ill and could no longer do those things.

After she left, the images changed. They became more specific, and a sentence began repeating inside my mind: You are going to get cancer.

I didn't tell many people because I knew how it sounded. There was no diagnosis, no suspicious scan, and no doctor warning me about anything. I wasn't experiencing a supernatural revelation that I could prove to anyone.

It was a thought, a fear, and a conviction I could not explain.

The darker I became emotionally, the stronger it felt. I began telling myself that I had to escape the death spiral or cancer would come. It felt as though the anger and despair inside me were turning into something physical, even though I understood there was no medical basis for making that connection.

I am not saying heartbreak causes cancer. I am not saying anger creates a tumor or that a person can prevent illness by thinking positively. People who develop cancer did not fail spiritually or emotionally, and I would never place that burden on anyone.

I am only describing what happened inside my mind. During the darkest period of 2020, I became convinced that cancer was waiting somewhere in my future.

The thought didn't make me suddenly grateful to be alive. It frightened me, but fear alone was not enough to pull me out. I remained trapped between not wanting to live and believing that a serious illness was approaching.

A few performances continued during the second half of 2020. Some couples moved weddings away from the cities and held them in barns, on private properties, or in mountain locations where gatherings could still take place. Those events gave us occasional work, although they did not restore the company.

Every show required more uncertainty than before. Rules varied by location, clients changed plans repeatedly, and nobody knew whether an event scheduled several weeks ahead would actually happen.

I also tried performing through the internet. Musicians everywhere were sitting in front of cameras and finding ways to reach audiences online. Some people became highly successful doing it, including performers I respected.

I probably completed around ten online shows, but the experience never felt natural to me. Dueling pianos depended upon interaction. I needed to hear people respond, watch them react, and adjust the show according to what was happening in the room.

Playing into a camera felt stale. I could see comments appearing on a screen, but I could not feel the audience. The energy that normally moved between us had been reduced to an internet connection.

I respected the people who found a way to thrive in that format, but I couldn't convince myself that it was the same thing. It kept music moving for a while, although it didn't restore the purpose I felt when standing in front of a live crowd.

Strangely, Sophie and Meg helped create one of the opportunities that arrived during that period. I posted a video of them eating their food and tagged the company that produced it. Somebody associated with the brand saw the video, began following what I did, and eventually contacted me about entertainment for a convention in Kansas City.

A simple video of my cats eating led to a paying event. After years of advertising, sales calls, and carefully edited promotional material, the absurdity of that was not lost on me.

The booking also reminded me that opportunities could arrive from places I had not planned. The company was damaged, but it was not dead. People still wanted what we did, even if the old routes toward reaching them had changed.

I began looking outside California for markets where live entertainment was returning more quickly. I had money available for marketing, and I decided to direct it toward Texas and Arizona rather than continue waiting for every California venue to reopen.

I hired a social media marketer to create a video that included my sobriety story and explained more about who I was and what The Killer Dueling Pianos represented. I had once tried to keep the business separate from the personal history behind it. Now I was beginning to understand that the history was part of the brand.

The company had been created through recovery. My experiences with addiction, leadership, failure, service, and rebuilding shaped the way I treated the performers and clients. Telling that story allowed people to see something beyond another entertainment act.

Venues in Texas began responding. Some were large rooms capable of holding approximately five hundred people, the kind of places that could help us establish recurring work. We developed opportunities at a place called Hambones in Palestine, another called Potosi Live in Abilene, as well as other cities like Temple and Gruver, and the calendar for 2021 gradually started filling.

The return didn't happen all at once. There was no single announcement that suddenly restored the company to what it had been before March 2020. Bookings appeared one at a time, often in different states and under conditions that continued changing.

Still, I could see movement. Performers who had barely worked for a year began receiving dates again, and the company started generating income.

I should have felt completely renewed. Instead, the external recovery of the business moved faster than my internal recovery.

I remained heartbroken. I could travel to a show, perform successfully, and then think about Red during the drive home. The fact that she had never contacted me remained difficult to accept.

Part of me continued expecting something. A message, an explanation, an acknowledgement of the five years we had spent together, or some indication that I had not simply been erased from her life would have been enough to prove the relationship had mattered to her.

Nothing came.

I had spent years learning how to accept situations I could not control, but acceptance did not mean approval or emotional indifference. It meant recognizing reality without continuing to destroy myself in an attempt to change it.

The reality was that Red had left and chosen not to speak to me again. I could not force closure from somebody who had decided not to provide it.

The pool was completed during this period. At first, I barely used it. I looked into the backyard and saw the same symbol of resentment that had been there during construction.

I swam a few times, but the experience felt connected to what the pool was supposed to have been. It was difficult to enjoy something I had purchased while begging another person to remain in my life.

Then I began experimenting with the controls and discovered the colored lights. At night, the water could shift through different colors and patterns, transforming the backyard into something completely different.

I turned them on and watched the pool change. For the first time, I found myself thinking that it looked pretty fucking cool.

That was a small moment, but it mattered. The pool had existed entirely as a reminder of Red, and now I had experienced something about it that belonged only to me. I had not installed the lights for her departure or for a future relationship. I had simply found something I enjoyed in my own backyard.

Gradually, I began reclaiming pieces of the house. It still contained memories, but not every object had to remain permanently attached to the relationship. The house could become mine, even if I had originally bought it while imagining us.

Sophie and Meg were already treating it that way. They had no concern for the meaning I attached to the mortgage, bedroom, pool, or furniture. To them, the house was where they lived with me.

Their certainty helped.

Early in 2021, I received a call from the Central Valley chapter of the Leukemia & Lymphoma Society. The woman for whom Donny and I had performed at the final fundraiser before the shutdown had become involved with the organization's board, and they wanted me to participate in the Man of the Year campaign.

The campaign required candidates to assemble teams and raise as much money as possible during approximately six weeks. Many of the people chosen were well established in the Central Valley. They had large families nearby, professional firms, hospital networks, fire departments, or businesses capable of producing major donations.

I was still relatively new to the area. The company had developed clients and friends there, but I did not have generations of relatives or a large corporate structure surrounding me.

When they asked, I became emotional. My immediate thought was that I had no idea how I could possibly do it. My piano players had barely worked for a year and were struggling financially. I could not ask them to carry a fundraising campaign when I was still trying to restore their income.

I told the organization that I would write a check for five thousand dollars and let that be my campaign. They encouraged me not to decide immediately and asked me to think about what might be possible.

I began making calls.

One of the first people I contacted was Bree Gentry, a previous client who had hired us for her own Woman of the Year campaign in 2017. She understood the process and told me not to worry. She would organize a fundraiser at her home and help create an event around our performance.

Her willingness to step forward surprised me. I had spent years believing that I needed to handle everything myself, but people were offering help before I had even learned how to ask for it properly.

The parents of another woman we had supported through a campaign also became involved. Her father told me to focus on rebuilding the company while they worked with the Lions Club to organize another event.

Other friends, clients, caterers, local businesses, and people throughout the Central Valley began contributing. Some donated money, while others offered food, space, labor, or whatever they could provide.

My parents donated. I reached out to relatives and longtime friends outside California. Dennis O'Brien, my best friend from childhood in Ohio, helped raise money from people who had known me long before The Killer Dueling Pianos existed.

Donny became my campaign manager. After everything he had already carried with me—the company, travel, the breakup, and the pandemic—he stepped forward again.

I named the team Ryan's Rockstars.

The name connected the campaign to music, but it also described the people appearing around me. The rockstars were not only the performers. They were the people opening their homes, organizing events, preparing food, calling friends, donating money, and deciding that I would not have to do the campaign alone.

For someone who had spent most of the previous year believing his life had no value, being surrounded by that level of support was overwhelming.

The campaign brought me back into active service. I was no longer raising money only to keep my own company alive. We were raising it for people fighting blood cancers, their families, and research that might give future patients more time.

That purpose reached a part of me that business success could not.

Halfway through the campaign, I looked at Donny and told him we were not finished with Ryan's Rockstars. I didn't know what the name would eventually become, but I felt that it had a purpose beyond those six weeks.

The campaign also brought Jennifer back into the center of my life.

Jen had died from acute myeloid leukemia, and more than fifteen years had passed since I had been in contact with her parents. I had continued praying to her throughout those years, but I had not known whether her family understood the role she still played in my life.

I contacted one of her relatives and asked whether her parents might allow me to dedicate the campaign to her. I wanted the money we raised to support research in Jennifer Stahl-Doyle's memory.

When word reached her mother, she apparently remembered me as "the piano player." That description brought me back to the version of myself who had known Jenn before sober living, before the company, and before so much of the life that followed.

I spoke with her parents through FaceTime. Tears ran down my face as I explained what I was doing and how often I had spoken to their daughter in my prayers. I told them that Jenn had continued inspiring me long after her death and that I wanted the campaign to honor her.

They gave me their blessing and told me they were proud of what I had accomplished.

Their words affected me deeply. When Jenn was dying, she had shown me a kind of courage and grace I did not understand. I had carried guilt over my own behavior, the years I lost to addiction, and the fact that I had been given time she did not receive.

Honoring her through the campaign did not resolve all of that, but it transformed part of the guilt into service.

Ryan's Rockstars raised approximately fifty-seven thousand dollars, all through private donations. We did not receive a large corporate check capable of carrying the campaign by itself. The money came from individuals, families, clients, friends, and community members who gave what they could.

I was not named Man of the Year. On the final night, we could not even attend because the company already had a show booked. I received the Big Heart Award instead.

More importantly, fifty thousand dollars of the fundraising success supported acute myeloid leukemia research in memory of Jennifer Stahl-Doyle.

The acknowledgement from the Leukemia & Lymphoma Society meant more to me than winning the title would have. Jen's name was connected to research that might help another patient survive the illness that had taken her.

For the first time in a long while, the pain inside me had become useful.

The campaign did not heal my heartbreak. I still thought about Red everywhere I went, and the blackness did not disappear simply because we had raised money for an important cause.

Service was not a cure. It was a reason to continue moving when I could not produce enough love for myself.

The campaign showed me that my life could still have value even when I didn't feel that value internally. The people around me had treated me as someone worth helping, and together, we had turned that help outward.

By the end of 2021, the company calendar was filling again. The Texas opportunities were growing, performers were returning to work, and The Killer Dueling Pianos had survived a collapse that once appeared capable of ending it completely.

My neighbors had become family. The house had begun feeling less like a monument to a failed relationship, and the pool no longer represented only resentment. Sophie and Meg remained beside me, as attached to me as I had become to them.

From the outside, I was recovering.

Inside, I still didn't feel whole. I remained sober, continued sponsoring people, worked the shows, and followed the opportunities appearing in front of me. I could recognize that I was helping people and feel grateful for everything returning to my life.

The black heart remained.

So did the premonition.

At some point during that period, I saw a billboard concerning head and neck cancer. There was nothing unusual about a medical advertisement, but the image seemed to demand my attention. I remember wondering why it felt so loud to me, as though it were speaking directly into the thought that had been following me since 2020.

The conviction returned: I was going to develop head and neck cancer.

There was still no medical evidence supporting that belief. Telling people would only have made me sound irrational, so I kept most of it inside and continued working.

The stages were returning. The company was rebuilding, and people were laughing again when Donny and I performed. Ryan's Rockstars had given Jennifer's memory a new form of service, and my neighbors had shown me that family could grow around a person in unexpected ways.

All of that was real.

The other feeling was real too. Somewhere beneath the bookings, gratitude, music, and service, I remained convinced that something was coming.

I didn't know when it would arrive or whether the fear had any meaning beyond the darkness of that period. I only knew that the thought would not leave me.

Cancer was waiting.

CHAPTER TWELVE

Something Isn't Right

"But it's fear, and you'll hear. It's calling you beware."

SONG: RAINBOW IN THE DARK.
BAND: DIO

Near the end of 2022 or the beginning of 2023, my father and I went over my bank accounts together. I had been so focused on the daily operation of the company that I had not stopped to calculate what everything added up to.

My father looked at the numbers and pointed out what should have been obvious. "Ryan, you're a millionaire."

I looked at the accounts again. This may not have been a big deal to most people, but the word felt strange when it was attached to me. I had spent years living from one performance to another, filing for bankruptcy, sleeping in a halfway house, renting rooms, and wondering whether I would ever have financial security.

Now the number was there.

"I'm a fucking millionaire," I said.

There was gratitude in that realization. I knew how fortunate I was, and I knew the money had not simply appeared. Donny, Johnny, Steve, the other performers, and I had worked for it. We had driven through the night, carried equipment into difficult venues, performed while exhausted, returned every call, chased every lead, and continued rebuilding after the pandemic nearly destroyed the company.

The money had not been handed to us. Every dollar represented years of work, although it also represented something else I was only beginning to recognize.

I had not slept properly in years.

I woke up and returned calls before doing almost anything else. Every inquiry seemed urgent because it might become a booking, and every booking might create more work for the people depending on the company. I chased leads, negotiated contracts, managed payroll, coordinated performers, solved equipment problems, and tried to remain available to everyone.

Donny worked with the same intensity. When he was not performing or driving, he was editing videos, developing promotional material, or working on some other part of the brand. Johnny and Steve were also carrying more responsibility, and the company continued expanding because all of us were willing to do far more than walk onto a stage and play songs.

The Killer Dueling Pianos had returned from the pandemic in a different form. Before 2020, people sometimes hired us because they wanted a dueling-piano show and happened to find our company. After the pandemic, more people began asking specifically for us.

They recognized the logo, the patch, the videos, the wine bottles, the performers, and the attitude behind the show. Donny and I were not rock stars in the traditional sense. We were not making records or hearing our songs on the radio, but inside the dueling-piano world, the company had developed a recognizable identity.

We traveled to Texas, returned to Ohio for shows, worked in Las Vegas, and flew across the country to several other states. The calendar became full again, and the money in the accounts continued growing.

Externally, I had reached a level of success I once believed would answer every question in my life. Internally, I was still asking the same question I had asked when the campaign ended.

Was this it?

I had the house, the pool, the company, the performers, the bank account, the motorcycles, the Mustang, and more work than I could accept. I could help people raise money through fundraisers and create employment for musicians I cared about. I was sober, sponsoring other people, and trying to live according to the spiritual principles that had saved me.

I could not reasonably complain about my life. I was living with an enormous amount of gratitude, but gratitude and emotional peace were not the same thing.

The heartbreak from Red's departure remained inside me. It was no longer as loud every day, but it had not disappeared. I could move through an entire week of shows without openly talking about it and still find myself thinking about her during a drive or after returning to the house.

Part of me continued judging myself by the fact that she had left. The success of the company had not changed the old belief that I was not enough. I could become financially secure and professionally respected, but some part of my mind still returned to the same conclusion: if I had been good enough, she would have stayed.

That conclusion ignored the complexity of the relationship and placed everything onto one person. I had made mistakes, lost my temper, and sometimes responded badly when I felt rejected. Red had her own reasons, choices, and emotional history. The relationship had not ended because of a single moment or a single failure.

I understood all of that intellectually. Emotionally, rejection was much simpler. It told me I had failed.

By 2023, I began trying to change the house so it no longer looked exactly as it had when Red lived there. My cousin Wendy encouraged me to repaint, remodel, hang things on the walls, and create an interior that belonged to me.

That process took time. Changing paint and furniture could not erase the past, but it could stop every room from remaining frozen in it. I began making decisions according to what I wanted instead of asking what Red would have preferred.

The house gradually stopped feeling like the scene of a relationship that had ended. It began becoming the place where I actually lived.

My neighbors helped with that process. Chris and Jenna and their daughters continued caring for Sophie and Meg whenever I traveled. They, and my other neighbors, put food in my refrigerator, checked on the house, and made sure the cats had what they needed.

My family remained deeply supportive, but they lived far away. I spoke to my parents and brothers, visited when I could, and never doubted that they loved me. My neighbors became a different kind of family because they were physically present in my daily life.

Chris became someone I could talk to about almost anything. He taught me about landscaping and helped me understand what I could do with the property. I had planted a lemon shrub in the backyard, and Chris built a pergola so the vines could grow around it.

Eventually, the plant produced more lemons than I could possibly use. The pool lights reflected across the backyard at night, the lemon tree continued growing, and the house began collecting memories that had nothing to do with Red.

I still did not celebrate Christmas there. The holiday remained too connected to 2019, the final Christmas before the business collapsed and the relationship ended. I could enjoy the house, but there were still parts of my old life I was not ready to reclaim.

The cats had already made the place theirs. Sophie and Meg had lived there long enough to understand every room, window, and hiding place.

They knew when I was packing for a trip and often began reacting before I carried anything to the vehicle.

When I was away, I checked the cameras inside the house and watched them move through their routines. Knowing that my neighbors were nearby made traveling possible, but I still missed the cats whenever I was gone.

They had been with me through the darkest period of my life. Caring for them had helped keep me alive when I did not see much value in my own existence, and the bond between us continued deepening.

The house, the cats, the neighbors, and the returning business should have made the premonition from 2020 disappear. Instead, the thought about cancer continued surfacing at unexpected moments.

During one of our trips to Bakersfield, I met a bar owner whose name was also Ryan. He had been through throat cancer and was on the other side of treatment.

The coincidence unsettled me. His name was Ryan, he worked around entertainment, and he had survived the exact kind of cancer that had somehow been living in the back of my mind.

I remember hearing his story and immediately thinking that I was going to get throat cancer too. Part of me wondered whether I already had it.

There was no rational reason for that conclusion. I had no diagnosis, no tumor, and no doctor suggesting anything was wrong. I knew how irrational it would sound if I told people that meeting a man named Ryan had confirmed a fear I had carried since the pandemic.

People would have told me I was being crazy, and they would have had a reasonable argument. The thought remained anyway.

I had already seen a billboard about head and neck cancer that seemed strangely loud to me. I had spent years participating in cancer fundraisers, and Jennifer's death remained part of my spiritual life. None of those things meant I was going to become sick.

My mind kept connecting them.

I did not want the book to present those experiences as proof that I predicted my own cancer. There was nothing medically significant about a billboard, a name, or an unexplained feeling. The power of those memories came later, after the diagnosis gave them a meaning they did not yet possess.

At the time, they were simply things I noticed and could not forget.

By 2024, the company was performing at a level that finally allowed me to relax slightly. We were still working constantly, but there was enough momentum behind the brand that I no longer felt every quiet week would destroy us.

Clients recognized us, repeat bookings continued, and new opportunities arrived through relationships we had spent years building. Donny and I had become identified with the company in a way I had once only imagined.

I was still working too much. Relaxing slightly for me did not mean taking long vacations or turning off my phone for days. It meant believing the business might remain alive if I stopped thinking about it for several hours.

That was progress.

I also began accepting that Red was not coming back. I didn't suddenly stop loving her or wishing the relationship had ended differently. I still hoped she was safe, happy, and living a life that met her needs.

The difference was that I could finally look at my own life and admit that it was not terrible. I had a nice home, a pool I had learned to enjoy, beautiful mountains nearby, extraordinary neighbors, a loving family, and a successful business.

Red was missing a good life, but I hoped she had found a good life of her own. I had wanted that for her even on the day she left.

My life continued moving, and early in 2024, a small gray cat started appearing outside my house.

He was young, mischievous, and immediately interested in me. He followed me around the neighborhood and began sleeping on the porch at night.

I put a bed outside for him but told myself I could not bring another cat into the house. Sophie and Meg had been living together for years and had developed a stable relationship. Introducing a young male cat could disrupt everything.

Meg had once been more closely attached to Red. After Red left, she became intensely attached to me. Sophie had her own connection with me, and both girls were comfortable with the house as it was.

I didn't want to disturb that balance.

The problem was that I was already falling in love with the gray cat. I named him Smokey and began checking the outdoor cameras whenever I traveled.

At night, I would look to see whether he was asleep on the porch. If he was not there, I checked repeatedly, waiting for one of the cameras to show that he had returned.

I worried that he would be hit by a car, attacked by another animal, or disappear while I was away. The amount of time I spent looking for him on the cameras made it obvious that I had already made an emotional commitment, even if I had not admitted it.

In May, something happened outside involving a very young child who did not understand how to treat the cat. The child struck Smokey, and that ended the debate for me.

I brought him into the garage, placed his bed, food, water, and litter box there, and called the veterinarian. I told them I was bringing in a cat and needed him checked.

The veterinarian tested him for diseases, looked for a microchip, and examined him. Smokey was healthy, had no chip, and appeared to be approximately nine months old. I had him neutered and received permission to bring him into the house.

When I took him out of the carrier after the procedure, the first thing he did was urinate all over my arm. I could not blame him. I would probably have done the same thing if someone had just cut my balls open and placed me inside a carrier.

It was approximately 108 degrees outside, but the stone floors inside the house were cold. Smokey came in, spread his legs, and lowered himself so the sore parts of his body could rest directly against the cool stone.

I had never seen him sit that way before, and I have never seen him do it since.

The humor helped, but the introduction to Sophie and Meg did not go well. Both girls hid for nearly two months, and I felt terrible that my decision had disrupted the home where they had felt secure.

Smokey was roughly their size when he arrived, but he was younger, male, and filled with energy. He wanted to play much more aggressively than they did, and they wanted almost nothing to do with him.

I had made the commitment, however, and I was not sending him back outside. He had chosen my porch, and by then, I had chosen him too.

Because Sophie and Meg avoided him, Smokey became more attached to me. He followed me through the house, grabbed my arm, rested his head against me, and remained close whenever I worked.

He was not afraid of music or noise in the same way the girls sometimes were. If I picked up a guitar or turned on an amplifier, Sophie and Meg might move somewhere quieter. Smokey stayed nearby.

His instincts were different because he had begun his life outside. He seemed to watch movement, sound, and human emotion in a way the other cats did not.

When I was traveling and looked through the cameras, I sometimes saw all three cats sitting near one another without a problem. When I returned home, Meg and Smokey competed for my attention and acted as though peaceful coexistence had never occurred.

The dynamic was imperfect, but the house now held three animals I loved. Smokey grew from a small gray cat sleeping on my porch into a sixteen-pound presence who seemed determined to involve himself in everything I did.

Later, I would attach enormous meaning to the way he watched me and reacted to changes in my body. At the time, I was simply grateful that he had found me.

During 2024, I also decided to join the Visalia Country Club. I had grown up around a country-club environment in Dublin, Ohio, so it didn't feel unfamiliar. The company had performed events there, and I already knew several members through business.

My main reason for joining was practical. I spent so much time traveling that I was rarely home long enough to shop, cook, and use the groceries before leaving again. The club would give me somewhere to have a good meal whenever I returned from the road.

I wanted to sit down, order something that tasted good, and avoid cooking for one person in a house where I might spend only two nights before the next trip.

The irony of joining a club partly because I wanted dependable, enjoyable meals would become obvious later. At the time, taste and swallowing were things I assumed would always be available to me.

Around October, while my membership application was still being processed, I began feeling something near my right tonsil. It felt as though a corn kernel or a piece of popcorn shell had become stuck there.

The sensation was not overwhelming. I could still work, travel, speak, sing, and eat. It was simply present often enough that I noticed it.

I looked into my mouth in the mirror. I had always had large tonsils, and I could not say exactly what was different. Something did not look completely right to me, but I was not a doctor and did not know what I was looking for.

My primary-care physician was dealing with his own cancer at the time, and I could not reach him easily. I went to an urgent-care clinic and tried to explain the sensation.

They told me I probably had COVID. I tested negative, but they still believed that was the likely explanation and gave me medication for it.

I knew what COVID felt like, and I did not believe that was what I had. I kept explaining that my throat did not simply feel sore. It felt as though something was stuck against my tonsil.

The sensation continued. In November, I returned to urgent care and tried again to explain what I was experiencing.

This time, they suggested strep throat. A nurse had written that I reported having a sore throat, but that was not what I believed I had said. I had described the feeling of a corn kernel against my tonsil.

They gave me antibiotics.

I took the medication, but I remained unconvinced. My body was telling me something, and the answers I was receiving did not match what I felt.

My country-club membership was approved the day before Thanksgiving. I went there for Thanksgiving brunch and was seated with a large family who treated me warmly.

I was alone, but I did not feel unwelcome. The environment reminded me of the world in which I had grown up, and being able to sit there represented how much my life had changed financially.

While eating, I felt the sensation in my throat again. Something seemed to catch or remain stuck near the tonsil when I swallowed.

The corn-kernel feeling had returned.

In the back of my mind, the old premonition became more specific. I thought about the billboard, the images from 2020, and the bar owner named Ryan who had survived throat cancer.

I began thinking that I had throat cancer.

I didn't know what throat cancer felt like. I had no medical evidence and no visible tumor. Two urgent-care visits had produced explanations that were far more common than cancer.

Still, I could not dismiss the thought.

December became one of the busiest periods of the year. Holiday parties filled the calendar, and there was little time to investigate a symptom that was annoying but had not stopped me from working.

That was how I had always handled physical problems. Musicians learn to perform through headaches, injuries, illness, exhaustion, and pain because the client has already gathered the audience and paid for the show.

The performance does not care how you feel. Neither does payroll.

I kept working.

Emotionally, I also began feeling that I might finally be all right. The business was doing well, and I had enough money to remain secure for a while. My neighbors continued supporting me, my family loved me, and Sophie, Meg, and Smokey had become the center of my home life.

Donny remained the hardest-working person I knew in show business. Johnny and Steve were doing exceptional work, and other players were ready to carry more responsibility.

I could look at my life without pretending Red was going to return. I still carried regret and heartbreak, but they were no longer the only things I could see.

Donny and I were hired to perform far out in West Texas for New Year's Eve. We completed the show and began traveling toward the airport on January 1, 2025.

During the drive, I looked at him and said, "I think I'm going to be okay."

Donny knew what I meant. We had spent years together on the road, and he had witnessed the depression and heartbreak that followed Red's departure. He had listened to the same thoughts more times than either of us could count.

For the first time, I believed I might be capable of accepting the life in front of me instead of comparing it with the one that had ended.

Then I added, "But something's not right."

Donny asked what I meant, but I didn't have a clear explanation I could give him. I only knew that the feeling in my throat and the conviction I had carried for years had not gone away.

I believed there was cancer inside me.

We returned from Texas on January 2. There were no immediate shows scheduled for the next few days, which gave me a rare opportunity to sleep and rest.

At approximately six in the morning on January 4, I woke up but did not want to move. Smokey had developed a habit of noticing the moment I was awake. If I shifted under the covers, he would come over and demand that the morning begin. If you have a cat, then you know this routine.

I remained still and pretended to be asleep.

Smokey came onto the bed. Normally, he might sit on my chest or try to get my attention. That morning, he began sniffing around my neck.

He sniffed one area repeatedly, gave it a small wet nose lick, and then placed his paw against my neck. He held it there for approximately five seconds, and then just walked away.

I continued lying still because I was pretending to be asleep, but I noticed how unusual the behavior was. Later, I joked with my parents and Donny that Smokey had taken my pulse.

At that moment, it was only a funny story about the cat.

Five days later, the lump appeared overnight.

On January 9, a mass seemed to pop out on the right side of my neck almost overnight. It looked like an enlarged lymph node, but I had never experienced anything like it before.

We had a show that night at Cal Coast Beer in Paso Robles, and the venue owner noticed the lump while talking with me. He didn't want to frighten me, but he told me I needed to have it examined.

I agreed. There was no doubt in my mind that something serious was happening.

People close to me tried to reassure me. Swollen lymph nodes were common. They could appear because of infections, viruses, or countless other things that were not cancer.

That might have been true for other people, but I knew my body. I didn't normally develop swollen lymph nodes, and this one had appeared after months of feeling something unusual near my tonsil.

My regular physician was still dealing with his own illness, and reaching him remained difficult. I began calling medical offices and imaging centers, trying to find someone who could examine the mass and order a scan.

Getting an appointment was much harder than I expected. The tumor was visible, but that did not automatically create urgency inside every office I contacted.

My friend Amber, a respiratory therapist living several hours away, tried to help me navigate the situation. She offered to connect me with an ENT near her if I couldn't get an appointment locally.

Eventually, I found an ENT in Visalia who could examine me. She placed a scope down my throat and said she didn't see anything obviously wrong.

The scope being clear should have reassured me. It didn't explain the mass in my neck.

I asked her to order a CT scan. She agreed, and I left believing the order would be sent to the imaging center.

The next day, I had not received a call. I contacted the imaging center and was told they had not received the order.

I called the ENT's office, and someone told me it had been sent. I called the imaging center again, and they said it had not arrived.

The same conversation continued for days. The ENT's office insisted the order had been transmitted, while the imaging center continued telling me it had received nothing.

By Thursday afternoon, there was still no order. On Friday morning, I left a message telling the office that I was on my way there and expected to receive the CT request when I arrived.

When I gave my name at the desk, one of the employees moved quickly into the back of the office. I asked the woman at the desk what was happening, and her reaction confirmed what I had begun to suspect.

The order had never been sent.

For several days, someone had continued claiming it had been handled rather than admitting the mistake. Meanwhile, I had a visible mass growing in my neck and no explanation for it.

They finally gave me the order. I called the imaging center directly and explained everything that had happened.

The normal wait could have been several weeks, but the people there understood the urgency and arranged an appointment for the following Tuesday.

By then, I had finally reconnected with my regular physician. I had the CT images sent to him so he could review them.

He did not initially believe the mass looked cancerous because it contained fluid, but he agreed that it needed further evaluation. He did refer me, though, to another ENT in Fresno.

The new ENT told me the tumor didn't belong in my neck. Communication between us was difficult, and I struggled to understand some of what he was saying through his mask and accent.

What I understood was that the mass could either be removed or left alone while we waited to see what happened. From my perspective, that was not a difficult decision.

If something didn't belong inside my neck, I wanted it taken out.

During those weeks, Dr. Chris Wray was following everything closely. Chris and I had known each other since I was fourteen, when we played music together in Ohio. He had become an anesthesiologist at UCLA, and even though cancer was not his medical specialty, he understood the system far better than I did.

I kept him informed about the appointments, imaging, and proposed surgery. He explained what he could and helped me understand what questions needed to be asked.

My family also knew what was happening. My parents and brothers followed the updates, although I tried not to frighten them unnecessarily while the doctors were still telling me the mass might not be cancer.

The people around me wanted to believe the reassuring explanations. I wanted to believe them too.

The problem was that I didn't.

The surgery was scheduled for March 19, 2025. The plan was to remove the tumor from the left side of my neck and send it to pathology.

The procedure turned out to be more complicated than simply removing a swollen lymph node. The tumor had coiled around my jugular vein and extended toward the base of my skull.

Even after the surgery, the ENT did not seem particularly worried that it was cancer. The mass contained fluid, and nothing in his tone suggested that I needed to prepare for a life-changing diagnosis.

He told me the tissue would be examined and that he would call me the following Monday to discuss the pathology. I did not need to return to the office for the results.

Five days after surgery, on March 24, I went back for a post-operative appointment. The drainage tube was removed, and the incision was checked.

I had approximately thirty stitches in my neck. They pulled whenever I swallowed, and the scar looked as though someone had tried to cut my throat.

I was not ready to return to the stage, but The Killer Dueling Pianos continued operating. The performers handled the scheduled shows while I managed what I could from home.

Contracts still required attention, clients still had questions, and payroll still existed. The surgery had interrupted my ability to perform, but it had not interrupted the business.

I waited for Monday's call.

On Friday, March 28, I was at home with the cats. The stitches were still in my neck, and I remained sore from surgery.

At approximately 3:30 that afternoon, a notification appeared from the hospital's online system. The pathology results had been released earlier than expected.

I opened the report.

The first line read, "Squamous cell carcinoma positive for p16."

The thought that had followed me through the pandemic, the billboard, the man named Ryan, the feeling near my tonsil, Smokey's paw against my neck, the lump, the scan, and the surgery had finally been given a medical name.

At that moment, the story caught up with the email that began this book.

I had known something was not right.

Now it was written in front of me.

CHAPTER THIRTEEN

The Last Shows

"What would you think, if tomorrow I was gone?"

SONG: UNDER THE MOON
BAND: B.RYAN MICHAELS

Once UCLA took over my case, the uncertainty changed shape. I no longer had to wonder whether I had cancer, but I now had to understand what everyone intended to do about it.

The diagnosis had arrived in an email on March 28. Within days, Chris Wray began moving my case toward UCLA, and on April 8, I met with the head of the ear, nose, and throat department there. I was told that under different circumstances, they might have performed a robotic tonsillectomy, but another surgeon had already opened my neck and removed the tumor. At that point, the priority was to determine the extent of the disease and begin treatment.

The incision from the surgery still needed time to heal. Once it did, I returned to performing because that was what I knew how to do. The diagnosis had changed everything emotionally, but I was not yet physically sick from cancer treatment. My voice still worked, my body could still carry equipment, and clients still had events scheduled.

For a few weeks, I existed in a strange space between being diagnosed and becoming visibly ill. I was a cancer patient, but I could still stand onstage and appear almost normal. People who did not know what was happening would have had no reason to suspect that a treatment team was preparing to aim radiation at my head and neck.

I started referring to myself as a cancer warrior. That language gave me something active to hold onto while I waited. I could not remove the cancer myself, but I could prepare to fight it, continue working, and try to make sure the company remained stable before treatment took away my ability to manage everything.

On April 28, Donny drove me to UCLA to meet the radiation oncologist, Dr. Ricky. The day had barely begun when the ordinary demands of my life began colliding with the medical ones.

UCLA called at eight that morning asking whether I had the CT scan performed in Visalia back in January. I had not known they needed it, so the hospital contacted the imaging center, and the imaging center contacted me for permission to release it.

Before nine thirty, I had already received seven work calls.

A client in Texas needed to reschedule July dates. Moving a performance was never as simple as choosing another night because we booked so far ahead. A client might offer another date, only for Donny, Tim, or the equipment already to be committed elsewhere.

I was trying to keep income flowing to the performers while also confronting the likelihood that I would be unavailable for much of the summer. The people in Texas were good to us and even offered to pay whether we found another date or not, but I still wanted to make the work happen.

Cancer had entered my life, but the company did not understand that it was supposed to stop calling.

Dr. Ricky spent approximately an hour and fifteen minutes with me. I was accustomed to medical appointments where someone spoke quickly, looked at a screen, and began moving toward the door before I had processed the first answer. This felt different.

He explained the treatment as thoroughly as he could. I would need additional imaging and something called a CT simulation. During that procedure, the team would make a mask designed specifically for my face, head, neck, and shoulders so that I could not move while the radiation was delivered.

The word mask immediately created anxiety, although I did not yet understand exactly what wearing it would feel like. I knew only that it would hold me still and that I had never done particularly well in confined medical machines.

I also needed a dental examination. I had not seen a dentist in almost nine years because I generally went only when something hurt, and nothing had hurt. The radiation team needed to know whether I had cavities, damaged teeth, or any condition that could create problems once treatment began.

Dr. Ricky explained that the radiation could affect my salivary glands, dry out my mouth, irritate my skin, and remove my sense of taste for six to nine months. A nutritionist would help me keep my weight up. If eating became difficult, I would rely on high-calorie shakes. If I lost too much weight or could no longer swallow, I might need to be fed through a tube.

None of that sounded pleasant, but my greatest concern was my voice.

I asked about it more than once. Music was not merely how I earned money. Singing was one of the first things that had ever made me feel useful, and it had remained part of my identity through addiction, sobriety, business failure, success, heartbreak, and the pandemic.

The idea of surviving cancer only to lose the ability to sing frightened me.

Dr. Ricky showed me where the radiation would be directed and where my vocal cords were located. He did not appear concerned that the treatment would destroy my voice. He said I might sound hoarse for a while, but he expected it to recover within several months.

Donny and I questioned him again because the answer mattered that much. Dr. Ricky remained confident.

Hearing that gave me my first genuine relief since the diagnosis. The treatment could damage many things, but the doctors did not expect it to take my voice.

The radiation technique was called intensity-modulated radiation therapy, or IMRT. As I understood it, the treatment could be shaped and directed more precisely toward the areas they needed to reach.

I would receive radiation five days a week for seven weeks. Chemotherapy would be given once a week, beginning on the same day as radiation. The chemotherapy was intended to make the cancer cells more responsive to the radiation.

Treatment was expected to begin around May 19 or May 20, although the date later became May 21. That gave me only a few weeks to perform, prepare the company, arrange somewhere to live near UCLA, and attempt to understand what my life would look like once the side effects began.

The doctors told me the survival rate for this cancer was approximately ninety per cent. That sounded encouraging, but percentages become less comforting when you are the person who has to occupy one side of them.

I wanted to be among the nine people who survived, not the one who did not.

My initial plan was to stay with Chris during the week. He had offered me space in Santa Monica so that I would not have to make the long drive from Visalia to UCLA every day. I hoped I might still drive home on weekends to see Sophie, Meg, and Smokey.

The doctors believed the first few weeks might be manageable. The last several weeks were expected to become much more difficult as the radiation accumulated.

I made one thing clear. Whatever my past with drugs and pain medication, I did not intend to suffer unnecessarily. I was not seeking intoxication. I was preparing to undergo treatment for cancer, and I wanted the pain controlled.

I spoke with my sponsor and members of my recovery circle during the drive home. They reminded me that receiving necessary medication for a life-threatening illness was not the same as returning to the behavior that had nearly killed me.

My friend, Roger Ducharme, also became a source of spiritual support. He was fighting multiple cancers of his own, and yet he continued calling to encourage me. We were scheduled to perform at Lorimar Winery in Temecula a few days later, and I hoped he would feel well enough to attend. Roger did attend our show. Sadly, Roger lost his battle with cancer that September.

The amount of support surrounding me was humbling. Donny was reorganizing his life around my appointments, Chris had guided me into UCLA, my neighbors were preparing to care for the cats, and people who had experienced cancer were offering whatever knowledge they possessed.

I kept asking why I had been given so much support when many patients faced the same disease almost entirely alone.

That evening, I still had another contract to type. Smokey lay beside me with his head resting on my wrist while I worked.

The following morning brought more contracts and a reminder that cancer was already shaping the future of the company. Several requested performances fell on dates when I would be receiving treatment. For the first time in years, I had to look at desirable work and admit that I probably could not be there.

I also learned that Mike Peters, the singer of The Alarm, had died after his own battle with cancer. The Alarm had been one of the defining bands of my teenage years. I had modelled parts of my high-school image after Mike and had covered the band's music with The Myst.

When I was sixteen, I saw The Alarm open for Pat Benatar in Columbus. Before the show, I encountered the band shopping in a store near the venue. I introduced myself and received their autographs. Mike Peters was the first real rock star I ever met, and he had been kind to an insecure teenage musician.

Now he was gone from cancer while I was preparing for my own treatment. The timing felt impossible to ignore.

Later that day, I contacted a seamstress in Visalia named Doreen Warren. She was well known in the local motorcycle community for sewing patches onto cuts, the sleeveless vests many riders wore.

I had purchased burgundy-and-white ribbons representing head and neck cancer and wanted them sewn onto mine. Until then, the diagnosis had existed in medical reports, appointments, and private conversations. Placing the ribbons beside the other patches on my cuts made the cancer part of my visible identity.

Doreen asked what the ribbons represented. When I told her I had recently been diagnosed with throat cancer, she nearly began crying.

She told me about her brother Dennis, a Vietnam veteran who had also gone through throat cancer. He survived that disease but later died from another condition, possibly connected to Agent Orange exposure.

I listened as she spoke about him and thanked her for sharing the story. I could have stayed there for hours. Cancer had begun connecting me with people in ways I had never expected, often through the memory of somebody they had loved.

When Doreen finished sewing the ribbons in place, I felt an odd sense of pride. I was not proud to have cancer, but the ribbons felt like a rite of passage. They announced that this was real and that I intended to face it openly.

The next morning, Donny and I left for four shows in four days. We would begin at The Cliffs in Pismo Beach, travel to Lorimar Winery in Temecula, perform at Rio Bravo Country Club in Bakersfield, and finish at a private birthday party near Los Angeles.

The clock was ticking down, and I knew these might be some of my last performances for months.

Before leaving Visalia, UCLA's speech and swallowing department called to schedule a swallowing-preservation consultation. Radiation could make swallowing increasingly difficult, and I might have to relearn basic movements that I had never considered before.

Taste, saliva, swallowing, chewing, and speaking had always happened automatically. Cancer was forcing me to study every ordinary function of my throat as though it were a skill I might lose.

At The Cliffs, I found a few minutes after sound check to walk down toward the beach. We had performed there several times, but I had never taken the time to walk to the water.

Touring was not a vacation. We usually arrived, unloaded, completed sound check, ate whatever was available, performed, packed the equipment, and left. Beautiful locations became backgrounds we barely noticed.

That day, I noticed.

The ocean felt different because I did not know when I would see it again. There was peace in recognizing that my schedule would soon slow down and fear in knowing why it had to.

Performing could function like a drug. The adrenaline, attention, and energy of an audience gave me something no quiet room could reproduce. I loved what I did, but I also believed entertainment served a purpose beyond my own need for applause.

People needed a few hours away from whatever burden they were carrying. They needed music, laughter, and permission to be distracted. I had been fortunate enough to make a living giving people that experience.

I told myself I would return to it after cancer.

The corporate show that night became the best event we had performed for that particular association. The crowd responded, the company delivered, and for a few hours, nothing about my life felt interrupted.

After the show, my new accountant emailed me about an eleven-thousand-dollar penalty the IRS claimed I owed. My accountant of nearly twenty years, Rick O'Connell, had died shortly before April 15 while attempting to resolve the issue.

Rick had first helped me when I was newly sober and nearly broke. His son Brian and I had lived in sober housing together, and he was my first roommate at the garage apartment in Hollywood. Brian recommended his father when I needed someone to prepare my taxes. The first time Rick handled them, he charged me almost nothing, $50.

As my life and business grew, the returns became more complicated, and his fee increased, but the relationship remained. Now he was gone, and the documentation proving the IRS had made an error appeared to have gone with him.

Cancer had not paused tax problems. It had simply become another problem competing for attention.

The next morning, Donny drove nearly five hours from Pismo to Temecula. During the trip, I had a video appointment scheduled with the hematology oncologist, Dr. Deborah.

I worried that the internet connection would fail if we attempted the call from a moving vehicle. Medical appointments already made me anxious because I did not know what questions I was supposed to ask. The possibility of losing the connection in the middle of an important explanation made it worse.

Roger and his wife, Celeste, lived in Menifee, so we stopped at their house and used their internet. Roger had been a supporter of the company since our early Temecula performances, and now both of us were dealing with cancer.

Dr. Deborah explained the chemotherapy and ordered another CT scan to confirm that my organs were healthy enough for treatment. She also explained that the chemotherapy drug could damage my hearing.

For a musician, that possibility was terrifying.

The proposed plan included another medication after chemotherapy that might help protect my hearing. At that stage, I did not completely understand the chemistry or timing. I knew only that one drug would help the radiation attack the cancer while another might reduce the damage created by the first.

I listened and asked questions, but eventually I had to accept that I was not a doctor or scientist. I could not redesign the treatment. My job was to understand what I could and show up.

Dr. Deborah made me feel that I would be cared for rather than processed. UCLA treated thousands of patients, yet the people speaking with me rarely made me feel like the next name on a schedule.

After the appointment, we continued to Lorimar Winery. Roger, Celeste, their son Chad, and Chad's girlfriend came to the show.

My friend Kristen Boano arrived with approximately twenty people. She had supported the company for years, hired us for a birthday celebration, sent cards, and checked on me after learning about the diagnosis.

John and Abby Westerman were also there. They had lost their twenty-year-old daughter Kirsten to leukemia and created an organization supporting young adults with cancer and the people trying to remain present for them.

Their experience immediately reminded me of Jennifer. John and Abby understood the importance of connection during illness because they had lived through what happened when a young person and family were forced to navigate cancer.

They had hired us for fundraisers before the pandemic and even created a drive-in event in 2020 where the audience listened through car radios and responded by flashing headlights and honking horns.

After my diagnosis, Abby had been one of the first people I called. Seeing them at Lorimar meant more than seeing familiar faces in the audience. They knew what cancer could take from a family, and they were still willing to stand beside someone beginning that journey.

The show went well, although my right hand was giving me serious trouble. The pointer finger I used to hold a guitar pick was swollen and painful. I did not know whether I had sprained it, torn something, or developed arthritis.

I hoped it would hold together until May 17, when I expected to play my final show before treatment.

The following day, we traveled to Rio Bravo Golf Club in Bakersfield. It was our first performance there, and I wanted the venue to become a repeat client.

UCLA called at approximately three thirty, just as we arrived to unload and prepare for sound check. The hematology-oncology team told me I needed a hearing test every week throughout treatment. They also needed to coordinate the medication intended to reduce hearing damage.

I was standing beside equipment in nearly ninety-degree heat while trying to schedule audiology appointments, communicate with a nutritionist, and understand changing treatment arrangements.

Donny continued unloading while I stepped away to manage the calls. The audiology department would call, then I would receive another message, and then someone else needed an answer. Every department had its own schedule, phone number, and reason why the matter needed immediate attention.

In the middle of that, Boeing contacted me about booking a show at the House of Blues in Anaheim on May 28.

A major client was requesting the kind of event I had spent years chasing, and I was standing in a parking lot trying to determine whether chemotherapy might damage my hearing.

That collision had become my life. One call concerned cancer, while the next concerned a show. I had to treat both as urgent because delaying a response could mean losing an appointment or a client.

Once the medical calls were settled, I returned Boeing's call, described our services, and sent preliminary information. I could not perform the event myself, but the company had other teams capable of carrying it.

That was one of the reasons I had built something larger than my own performances. The business could continue even when I could not stand onstage.

At Rio Bravo, the floor plan was not arranged in the way I believed would best support the show. I hesitated to say anything because it was our first time at the venue and I did not want to appear difficult.

I had performed thousands of dueling-piano shows, however, and I knew that a poor layout could damage the audience's experience. Protecting the show sometimes required speaking up even when doing so made me uncomfortable.

The staff listened and rearranged the patio despite the heat. Their willingness to trust my experience told me what kind of people they were.

The performance became a success, and they wanted us to return twice a year.

During the evening, I spoke with Kim, one of the venue owners, who had worked with cancer patients for more than a decade. I told her how much anxiety I felt over the upcoming MRI.

Six years earlier, I had attempted an MRI and could not finish it. I remembered being pulled out of the machine and feeling humiliated by the reaction of the technicians. Whether they had intended to mock me or not, the experience remained inside my body as trauma.

I could tolerate CT and PET scans, but the MRI felt different. The confined space triggered intense claustrophobia, and I had begun having panic attacks merely thinking about it.

The fear was not only of the machine. I was terrified that I would panic, waste everyone's time, and delay the treatment intended to save my life.

I could stand before thousands of people, sing the wrong note, and recover. I could handle difficult clients and equipment failures. The thought of being trapped inside that machine reduced me to someone who could not sleep.

Dr. Ricky had prescribed Ativan, but I did not believe the amount would be enough. Asking for more help created another kind of fear.

Since childhood, I had carried the belief that I was an inconvenience. I worried that I was in the way, asking too much, or disturbing someone who had more important things to do. Nearly twenty years of sobriety had not completely removed that feeling.

Part of me worried that Dr. Ricky wouldn't comprehend my anxiety. Another part knew that hiding the truth would create a much larger problem.

After speaking with Kim and Donny, I wrote to him. I explained the previous failed MRI, the panic attacks, the fear of delaying treatment, and the possibility that I needed deeper sedation.

I was awake at one in the morning writing that message because the anxiety had become impossible to contain. I told him that I needed to be put under or placed into some form of twilight sedation.

Then I ended the night thinking about how much I missed my cats.

The fourth show of the run was a birthday party in Montebello. I slept until after noon because my body needed the rest.

We performed for approximately two and a half hours. During the final hour, the area around my tonsil hurt badly. It felt as though a large popcorn kernel remained stuck in my throat.

The sensation that had begun months earlier was no longer subtle.

Afterward, I drove home long enough to handle payroll deposits, taxes, household chores, and a few hours with Sophie, Meg, and Smokey.

I would soon have to return to Los Angeles for more scans and appointments.

Smokey bounced through the house when I arrived. Being able to pick him up, smell his fur, and feel his weight against me brought an immediate comfort I could not find anywhere else.

Sophie and Meg were accustomed to my traveling, but they still responded when I came home. All three cats had their own way of making the house feel inhabited.

My neighbors continued showing up too. Chris pruned the lemon shrub because he knew I might not have time or energy to do it later.

KC and members of his family came down the street carrying biscuits and freshly cut watermelon. We began talking in the garage about the treatment, and the men placed their arms around me and prayed.

Receiving prayer affected me more than I expected. I had spent decades learning how to provide for others, perform for strangers, and manage employees. Allowing people to stand around me and ask God to protect my life required a different kind of surrender.

I told them the cancer itself did not frighten me as much as asking for help. Depending upon others meant accepting that I could no longer control everything.

KC's young son saw the tears in my eyes and walked over to hug me. He might not have understood the reason for the emotion, but he understood that somebody needed comfort.

Later that evening, I recorded a video publicly announcing my diagnosis. Until then, only part of my professional and personal circles knew. Posting the video meant surrendering control over who received the information and how they reacted.

The response was enormous. Messages, calls, and prayers began arriving from people in different periods of my life.

I was grateful, but receiving that amount of care was almost uncomfortable. The old part of me still believed good things were meant for somebody else.

The following morning, Dr. Ricky called personally. He told me that the MRI was not essential. It might provide additional information, but the other scans gave him what he needed to plan the treatment.

He was willing to bypass it rather than force me through an experience creating that much psychological distress.

The relief was immediate. More important than the canceled test was the fact that he had listened. He did not dismiss the fear, lecture me about controlling my anxiety, or make me feel weak.

He also reassured me again that the treatment was not expected to destroy my voice. His confidence did not eliminate every fear, but it gave me something concrete to hold onto.

The nutritionist called later that day. She explained that I could eat almost anything before treatment, but chemotherapy days might require small, bland meals such as rice, bananas, or toast. I needed to remain hydrated and avoid foods that might burn or irritate the throat once the side effects began.

By the fourth week, eating could become extremely difficult. She did not know exactly how my body would react because treatment affected every patient differently.

That uncertainty appeared in nearly every conversation. Nobody could tell me precisely when food would stop tasting normal, when swallowing would become painful, or how much weight I might lose. They could describe what often happened, but they could not tell me exactly what would happen to me.

Kim continued bringing food to the house. She had been a friend for a long time, and now it was as if I was a project she was committed to completing.

I spoke with my parents through FaceTime and tried to explain the growing schedule of tests and appointments. My father had survived prostate cancer, and both of my parents understood that encouraging statistics did not remove fear.

They were too old to travel across the country easily. I did not know when I would see them again, and Mother's Day was approaching. The distance felt much greater now that I was preparing for treatment.

I went to dinner at Visalia Country Club. 2 of the servers there, David and Celini , asked how I was doing. The staff there knew I was waiting for results. I told them I had cancer. They both immediately gave me hugs, and David made sure I had his number and told me to call him 24/7 if I needed anything.

That night, Kristen Cady, another dueling-piano performer living with cancer, called and gave me practical advice about chemotherapy. She suggested preparing a bag with a blanket, eye covering, neck pillow, and anything else that might make the hours in the infusion chair more tolerable.

These were things no medical explanation had made me consider. Cancer survivors knew details that people learned only by sitting in the chair themselves.

The next day, I returned to Los Angeles for a chest CT ordered by Dr. Deborah. Donny dropped me near the UCLA building, and the scan was finished before he managed to park.

On the way back to his house, six new contract requests arrived. I liked booking shows, but writing contracts required a type of concentration that did not come naturally. My mind wandered, especially now that medical appointments occupied so much of it.

Still, each completed contract created a small sense of accomplishment. It meant the company was continuing to move.

That evening, I received a message from Rob Stichweh, a childhood neighbor I had not spoken with in years. Our families had lived beside each other in Dublin, and Rob, his sister Betsy, and I had grown up riding bicycles, skateboarding, swimming, fishing, and attending neighborhood pig roasts. We were family.

Rob had seen the announcement about my cancer. He told me that he was a year into remission after stage-four colorectal and liver cancer. Betsy had recently completed treatment for stage-three colon cancer and was doing well.

We spoke for approximately an hour. He did not attempt to tell me which medical choices to make, but he advised me to receive regular hydration during treatment.

More than anything, the call returned me to a time before addiction, business, and cancer. We remembered the neighborhood our parents had created for us and the freedom we had as children.

I did not fully appreciate that childhood when I was living it. Hearing Rob's voice reminded me how fortunate we had been.

The following morning, Donny and I returned to UCLA for the CT simulation. This was the appointment where the radiation team would build the mask.

A nurse suggested I take the Ativan that had originally been prescribed for the MRI. I agreed, although the procedure did not turn out to be as frightening as I expected.

The staff brought humor into the room immediately. I asked whether they needed to cut my hair to make the mask work, and one of the technicians joked about whether I wanted her to cut it.

We decided that the hair could be pulled through the top of the mask instead. I did not need to shave my head.

They formed a warm, molded pillow around the back of my head. When it did not feel comfortable, I forced myself to say something.

The staff did not act inconvenienced. They simply started again and created another one.

That small interaction mattered. Cancer was teaching me that advocating for myself did not automatically make me difficult. I could speak up without apologizing for needing to be comfortable.

The mask itself was made from a mesh-like material pulled tightly over my face. A bite guard was placed between my teeth, my eyes remained closed, and the material gradually hardened into the shape of my face and head.

As it dried, the pressure increased. I could feel the mask becoming heavier even though it was only tightening around me.

The longest portion lasted approximately ten minutes. While they formed the mask, the team moved me through the CT machine and gathered the images needed to plan the radiation.

I survived the process partly by doing what I always did. I made jokes.

When one technician asked how the pressure felt, I said it felt like someone had been sitting on my face, which was coincidentally how I got this cancer in the first place.

The staff burst out laughing.

The cancer was related to HPV, which in this case was transmitted through oral sex. Pretending otherwise would not change it. If I could not find humor in what was happening, the disease would take more than my health.

I told them that if I could not have fun with cancer, they could have it back.

The jokes were not denial. I knew the treatment could become brutal. Humor allowed me to enter a frightening room without surrendering every part of myself to fear.

After the simulation, we hurried to the audiology department. Because cisplatin could damage hearing, the team needed a baseline and planned to test me every week.

The results showed that I already had moderate hearing loss and qualified for hearing aids. Years of loud stages, amplifiers, speakers, and live performance had already taken a toll.

The audiologist advised me to avoid loud environments during treatment. That meant I might not be able to attend company shows even on days when I felt physically strong enough.

Hearing was as central to my musical life as my voice. I could adapt to many changes, but the possibility of losing the ability to hear pitch, music, and the people around me was difficult to accept.

From audiology, we went to the dentist. I had no dental insurance and expected that nine years away from a dental chair might produce an expensive list of problems.

The assistant took eighteen X-rays. The dentist examined my teeth, gums, tongue, lips, and throat, looking for anything that might interfere with radiation.

To my amazement, my teeth were fine. There were no new cavities, cracked teeth, or damaged fillings that needed to be repaired before treatment.

The appointment cost $338. That was my total dental expense for nearly nine years, which felt like a rare victory.

Two days later, my UCLA calendar changed almost instantly. Approximately thirty appointments appeared before noon. On some days, three or four appointments were scheduled across eight or ten hours.

Staying with Chris had initially seemed practical, but traveling between his condo and the hospital throughout the day would become complicated and expensive. Friends who had received care at UCLA recommended the Tiverton House, a hotel serving patients and located within walking distance of the medical buildings.

The hotel would allow me to keep my car nearby, avoid daily hospital parking, and return to the room during gaps between appointments. The rooms had two beds, which meant someone could stay with me without sharing mine.

I decided to reserve a room for the seven weeks of treatment. I hoped I could still return to Visalia on weekends, but I wanted the room available even if I became too sick to travel.

The cost would be approximately seven thousand dollars out of pocket. I had wanted to take a vacation that year, but comfort during cancer treatment became the vacation budget.

That afternoon, Donny and I performed at Engelmann Cellars. The winery had become one of the most important venues in the company's Central Valley history. Bret and Elainea Engelmann had supported us for years and even created several wines carrying The Killer Dueling Pianos label.

The property was surrounded by farmland, and the sunsets seemed worth more than anything money could buy. It had become one of the few places where I consistently felt at peace.

That night, I tried to absorb everything. I watched the sunlight disappear, noticed the sky darkening over the fields, and breathed as though I could store the atmosphere somewhere inside me.

We already had another performance scheduled there in August, but I knew I might not be ready. I told Bret I hoped he would book us again for 2026 because I wanted to return like a rock star.

It was also my father's eighty-seventh birthday, with Mother's Day two days away. My parents had never been able to see the home, neighbors, or Central Valley community that had become central to my life.

During the performance, I asked the audience to sing happy birthday to my father and wished my mother a happy Mother's Day.

After the show, Mike Junior from the sound crew asked whether he and several of the men could pray over me. I accepted immediately.

When Donny and I returned home, I jumped into the pool to wash away the sweat and grime. The temperature had reached approximately ninety-five degrees, and the water felt good.

I did not expect to swim during treatment because of the risk of infection and the need to protect my skin. Missing the pool seemed like a small sacrifice if the treatment saved my life, but I had only recently learned to love it.

The next morning, a letter from the insurance company was waiting in the mailbox. They had refused to cover the medication intended to reduce the risk of hearing damage from cisplatin.

The letter stated that the drug was not approved for an adult with my type of neck cancer. I could appeal, remain on hold, file a grievance, or hire someone to fight the decision. The cost per dose was $40,000, and I would need 7 doses.

Treatment was beginning in a matter of days.

I had said from the beginning that I did not want to spend whatever time I had left arguing with an insurance company. I had watched friends lose years of their lives to cancer and bureaucracy at the same time.

The denial sent me immediately back into the darkest part of my mind. I threw my phone across the kitchen and began questioning whether I wanted treatment at all.

I was not afraid of death in the same way I was afraid of prolonged suffering, stress, and losing the parts of myself that made life recognizable. I did not want to survive only to spend years fighting institutions while unable to hear, sing, play, or work.

Then I saw Smokey sitting on the kitchen counter. I wrapped my arms around him and began sobbing.

I did not want to leave my cats. I did not want to put that loss onto my family either.

I contacted my brothers, Dr. Deborah, Chris, and anyone who might know of another option. My brothers Rick and Sean found information about organizations that might help with the cost. Sean spoke with me long enough to pull me away from the edge of giving up.

Chris reminded me that specialists often knew ways to obtain approval or adjust treatment. Brad, another sober friend who had survived the same cancer, spoke with me for approximately an hour and described some of what might lie ahead.

Brad used the phrase "surrendered to win." It was an idea I understood from recovery. Sometimes continuing required admitting that my preferred plan was gone and accepting the help or circumstances in front of me.

I still had to leave for a fundraiser in Santa Maria. The client and audience did not know the insurance letter had nearly convinced me to abandon treatment.

The fundraiser supported a high-school student raising money for classmates who needed help attending a private Catholic school. The show took place in a gymnasium, the kind of room that could either succeed beautifully or become an acoustic disaster.

That night, it worked. The crowd was generous, Donny was exceptional, and I lost myself in the performance.

For a few hours, the anger disappeared because the music was helping someone I might never meet.

When I returned home, two more insurance envelopes were waiting.

That was the rhythm of those weeks. A show might lift me into gratitude, and the mailbox could pull me back into fear before I entered the house.

The IRS continued demanding the eleven thousand dollars my late accountant had been disputing. The newest letter threatened to freeze accounts and income.

I finally paid the money. I did not believe I owed it, but I could not fight cancer while worrying that the government might interfere with the accounts supporting the company.

My new accountant believed he could eventually recover it. At that moment, paying was the fastest way to remove one emergency from my life.

The ordinary world kept producing strange reminders of mortality. While renewing vehicle registration, an employee asked whether I wanted a life-insurance quote.

I had no wife or children, and enough money existed to cover funeral expenses. Still, the question forced me to think about estate planning and what would happen if treatment failed.

At the same time, a stray black cat in the neighborhood had given birth to kittens and moved them into Chris's garden. I visited several times a day to watch them.

Their mother trusted me more than most people, and I sat near the kittens as the sun went down, wondering whose lives those animals might one day save.

In the middle of planning for death, I was watching new life begin beside my house.

The final three shows arrived quickly.

The first was a public performance at Barrel House in Visalia. We had not played many public local shows since the company became widely recognized, and more than two hundred tickets were sold for a Thursday night.

Friends from across the Central Valley attended. Kim was there, Julie Estrada drove from Paso Robles, and neighbors and longtime supporters filled the room.

The performance became one of the strongest public shows we had played in the area. For a few hours, I was not preparing to become a patient. I was simply doing what I had spent my life learning to do.

My hands hurt badly. Holding a guitar pick had become difficult, and I did not know whether the problem was arthritis or another injury. Cancer had not caused every physical problem in my body, but the timing made each one feel more threatening.

The next day, we traveled into the Sierra Nevada mountains for a fundraiser at the Shaver Lake Museum. The outdoor amphitheater sat among tall trees at approximately 5,500 feet, with a large gray rock behind the stage.

The crowd numbered around 130 people, but the space felt full. It took several songs for my voice to warm up, and then the familiar feeling returned.

The magic was still there.

Donny performed as brilliantly as he always did, and the audience responded quickly. Before the night ended, the organizers wanted to book us as the opening act for the next year's concert season.

I told them to reserve the date immediately. I wanted an appointment on the calendar with the future.

Back at my house, Johnny, Steve, and Julie joined Donny and me. We stayed awake talking, laughing, and playing with Smokey.

Johnny and Steve had traveled from Southern California to handle another fundraiser the following day. Four Killer Dueling Pianos events would occur across California that weekend.

The company I once feared could not survive without me was now proving that it could.

Before leaving for our final performances on May 17, I took Donny, Johnny, and Steve to lunch at the country club. I thought of it as a metaphorical last supper while I could still chew, swallow, and taste normally.

They worked with me and technically worked for me, but underneath the business structure, they were my closest friends. Having them around before treatment meant more than I could explain.

Johnny and Steve left for a fundraiser in Lemoore. Donny and I drove to Kingsburg for a birthday celebration hosted by longtime supporters Alan and Kelly Roberts.

The wind was strong, and cigar smoke moved through the outdoor air. My anxiety turned every particle into a possible infection that could delay treatment.

I wondered whether a sinus infection, bronchial problem, or ordinary illness might prevent me from beginning on time. Before cancer, I would have ignored all of it. Now every physical sensation carried the potential to interfere with the schedule.

The final two songs requested that evening were "Let It Be" and "Don't Stop Believin'." The choices felt appropriate, even though nobody had planned them as a farewell.

When the performance ended, I wanted to stay and spend time with our friends, but my body and mind were exhausted. Treatment had not even begun, and the preparation alone had drained me.

Someone asked how I was doing. I had reached the point where the simplest answer was the most accurate: I had cancer, and that was about it.

There was no way to wish it away or return to the day before the diagnosis. The treatment was coming, whether I felt ready or not.

I imagined myself inside a landing craft approaching a beach under fire. The door would eventually fall open, and I would have to move forward into something designed to hurt me in the hope that it would destroy the cancer first.

People continued saying I would be fine. I wanted desperately to believe them, but nobody could guarantee the result.

The night ended with me telling myself that I would sing again.

For the next thirty-six hours, I wanted only to remain close to the cats.

Before leaving Visalia, I put many of the guitars from the living room into a locked closet. The room looked strangely organized without them.

I typed contracts, washed dishes, completed laundry, cleaned the house, and tried to prepare everything as though I were leaving for another tour. The routine was familiar, but the reason was not.

I told Sophie, Meg, and Smokey repeatedly that I loved them. They had experienced my absences before, sometimes for weeks, but this departure felt different because I did not know what condition I would be in when I returned.

My neighbors would care for them. I trusted that completely. What frightened me was not whether the cats would be fed. It was how much I needed to see them again.

Dave Harris, a friend from the Columbus music scene, answered after we had gone many years without a real conversation. Hearing his voice brought me back to another period of my life, before either of us knew what the future would demand.

Old friendships kept appearing at the exact moments I needed them. Cancer had begun reopening parts of my past while making the future uncertain.

Before leaving my house, I took my chopper for one final ride through Visalia. I wanted to feel the wind against my face and watch the sun go down from the motorcycle before treatment made riding impossible.

When I arrived at the Tiverton House, I checked into Room 152. It looked like an ordinary hotel room, but I had never entered a hotel under circumstances like these.

Most of my hotel arrivals followed performances. I usually entered carrying leftover adrenaline, talking about the crowd, and preparing to sleep for a few hours before the next drive.

This time, I was checking in for the battle of my life.

Living in Visalia had changed me. Los Angeles traffic, tall buildings, and the density of the city made me uncomfortable. I had become accustomed to open skies, mountains, neighborhood streets, and the ability to see the sun.

The Tiverton was close to UCLA, which was the point. I reminded myself that proximity to the hospital mattered more than comfort with the city.

A large grocery store stood across the street. I walked through aisles filled with fresh food, drinks, desserts, and many of the things I enjoyed eating.

Then I remembered that within weeks, I might be unable to taste or swallow most of them.

I purchased yogurt, protein shakes, drinks, food for the room, and plastic utensils. When I was alone, I expected to eat simply and avoid restaurants.

The room contained a small refrigerator but no freezer. I had been given special ice gloves and socks intended to reduce the risk of neuropathy during chemotherapy, but they needed to be frozen overnight.

The communal freezer was already full, so Donny and I began searching for a small freezer we could keep in the room.

Even the simplest preparations produced unexpected complications. Cancer treatment required appointments, medication, transportation, housing, food, cooling equipment, documents, and enough organization to maintain all of it while becoming increasingly sick.

The hotel also required a letter confirming that I would receive long-term treatment. Guests were generally limited to twenty-nine days, but the social worker helped obtain documentation allowing me to remain through July 19.

That approval gave me one less thing to worry about.

Before treatment began, I had breakfast with Johnny and Steve. Donny had already left temporarily to deal with work, and I spent the remainder of the day preparing the house, speaking with my family, and trying to accept that the start date had finally arrived.

I told my parents that the encouraging statistics did not completely comfort me. When the tumor appeared, nearly everyone believed it was unlikely to be cancer. The doctors had seemed unconcerned until the pathology proved otherwise.

I had been right about that, which made it difficult to surrender completely to anyone saying I would be fine.

I wanted my parents to understand that my jokes did not mean I had ignored the possibility of dying. Humor was how I moved through fear. It was not proof that fear was absent.

Jamie McNeill called that night. We spoke for approximately forty minutes about our friendship and the bond created through the patch. I had expected to perform with her again at Sturgis in August, but I knew that was unlikely.

I told myself we would do it in 2026.

The day before treatment started, I met with the speech pathologist for swallowing preservation. She taught me exercises intended to keep my tongue, throat, and neck muscles working even if my diet became entirely liquid.

I had to press my tongue against the roof of my mouth, hold it there, repeat neck movements, and practice forceful swallows. If the muscles weakened too much, I could remain dependent on a feeding tube long after treatment ended.

These exercises were now part of my job. I understood repetitive behavior, and I intended to perform them as often as necessary.

I met Chris for lunch before he left town for two weeks. I looked at the man I had known since I was fourteen and considered everything that had brought us to that table.

We had once been teenagers making music in Ohio. Forty years later, he had helped guide me into the hospital system that might save my life.

I did not know where I would be without him.

Throughout the afternoon, I called my parents again and responded to friends sending final messages before treatment. I typed a wedding contract for 2026 and sent instructions for the company events scheduled that weekend.

The future remained on the calendar even as I prepared to enter something that could change all of it.

Donny stayed in Room 152 with me that night. We set the alarm for 5:30 in the morning.

Chemotherapy was scheduled for seven. My first radiation treatment would follow at one that afternoon.

There was nothing more to prepare, nothing left to research, and no additional show I could perform before it began. The contracts were sent, the teams knew their assignments, the cats were being cared for, and the mask was waiting at UCLA.

I had spent the previous weeks saying goodbye to stages, friends, food, the pool, the motorcycle, my house, and the ordinary use of my own body. I did not know which of those things would return exactly as they had been.

What I knew was that the waiting had ended. In a few hours, the treatment would begin.

Donny and I turned in for the night with the alarm set beside us.

It was time to get it on.

CHAPTER FOURTEEN

Bolted to the Table

"Mm, get high with a little help from my friends."

SONG: WITH A LITTLE HELP FROM MY FRIENDS
BAND: THE BEATLES

The alarm went off at 5:30 on the morning of May 21. Donny, Kim, and I took the hotel shuttle to the hospital at six, arriving early enough that the doors to the department were still locked.

We waited downstairs until someone let us in. There was no dramatic entrance or ceremonial beginning to treatment. We sat inside a hospital before most of the building had fully opened, waiting for the chemicals and radiation intended to save my life.

I had spent the previous weeks preparing for that morning. The appointments had been scheduled, the mask had been made, the hotel room was stocked, and the company's performers knew which shows they were covering. My cats were being cared for in Visalia, and everyone around me had said whatever they believed might encourage me.

None of that changed the fact that I had never received chemotherapy before. I did not know what it would feel like as the drugs entered my body or whether I would experience an immediate reaction.

When the department opened, a technician brought me into the chemotherapy suite and placed me in a comfortable chair. Only one person could remain beside me, so Donny and Kim took turns.

The nurse inserted an IV into my arm. The first bag contained potassium chloride, dextrose, and sodium chloride. As I understood it, the mixture provided fluids and electrolytes before the chemotherapy began.

That portion took approximately two hours. Afterward came dexamethasone, a steroid, and fosaprepitant, which I understood to be intended to prevent nausea.

Eventually, the nurse hung the cisplatin.

After all the warnings about what chemotherapy could do, the drug entered quietly. There was no dramatic physical reaction and no immediate sense that something dangerous was moving through me.

I could stand up, walk to the restroom, use my phone, and work on my laptop. The chair was comfortable, and the staff checked on me regularly.

Four hours might have felt like a long time to somebody unaccustomed to sitting still, but Donny and I had spent years riding together in trucks between performances. We knew how to exist in one place for hours while answering calls, discussing shows, and trying to remain productive.

For a while, I thought chemotherapy might be manageable. I could imagine bringing the laptop each week and handling contracts while the drugs entered my body.

The nurse told me that the dosage was lower than some chemotherapy regimens. At that stage, it appeared I might not need the frozen gloves and socks I had purchased to reduce the risk of neuropathy, and I was not expected to lose my hair.

That was reassuring, although I already understood that keeping my hair did not mean keeping everything else. The treatment could still damage my hearing, taste, saliva, swallowing, nerves, and ability to perform.

None of that happened during the first few hours. I sat in the chair, talked with Donny and Kim, and allowed myself to believe that the medical part might be less frightening than the anticipation had been.

When the chemotherapy finished, Donny and I walked back to the Tiverton. I changed clothes, drank some water, and prepared to return to the hospital for radiation.

The chemotherapy had taken most of the morning. Radiation was scheduled for one that afternoon, which gave me only a short break between the two.

My heart rate was elevated when we returned to the hospital. I did not know whether the cause was the walk, the steroid, the chemotherapy, or anxiety. It was probably some combination of all four.

The radiation table was waiting in the treatment room, along with the mask that had been molded to my face two weeks earlier. During the simulation, I had managed to joke with the staff while the material hardened around me. The actual treatment felt different because I knew they would bolt the mask to the table and leave the room.

Tim and Kevin were the radiation technicians that day. They were calm and patient from the moment I entered.

I lay down while they positioned my head and pulled my hair through the opening at the top of the mask. The bite guard went into my mouth, and the mesh came down over my face.

As the mask tightened, my mouth became dry. I felt the need to swallow, but the bite guard and pressure around my neck made every movement feel restricted.

My anxiety began climbing quickly.

Tim and Kevin did not rush me. When I told them I needed to sit up, they released me, allowed me to rinse my mouth, and waited until I was willing to try again.

I returned to the table and attempted to focus on my breathing. The Rolling Stones played through the speakers, and I tried to use the music the same way I had used it throughout my life.

The difference was that music normally gave my body somewhere to move. On the radiation table, I had to remain completely still.

Once the mask was secured, I could not speak. The bite guard occupied my mouth, and the material held my face tightly enough that communication became almost impossible.

My hand remained free, so I raised it with my thumb and fingers extended. I was not signaling for them to stop. I needed somebody to understand that I wanted human contact before they left the room.

Kevin understood.

He walked over, took my hand, and placed his other hand around it. It was the kind of grip Donny and I might have exchanged after a performance, part handshake and part reassurance.

That handshake saved my soul.

My anxiety had been seconds away from becoming uncontrollable. Kevin did not offer a speech or tell me that there was nothing to fear. He held my hand long enough for me to understand that another person was still there.

Both technicians told me I was doing well and that the procedure would be over soon. Then they left the room to operate the equipment.

The table moved, and I heard the machine taking its initial images. I concentrated on remaining still and thought about Jennifer and my cats.

I did not know whether the timing meant anything, but "Sympathy for the Devil" began playing just as the machine started delivering the radiation.

The coincidence was so perfectly dark that part of me wanted to laugh. There I was, bolted beneath a mask while radiation entered my neck, listening to Mick Jagger introduce himself as Satan.

My sense of humor was still present, but it could not remove the fear. I worried that swallowing at the wrong moment or moving my head slightly would cause the radiation to strike somewhere it was not supposed to go.

The mask made meaningful movement almost impossible, but anxiety did not care about that fact. My mind insisted that I could ruin my own treatment through one involuntary swallow.

Postnasal drainage continued moving into my throat. The instinct to swallow was automatic, and fighting it made me feel as though I might choke.

I remained on the table until the machine stopped. When the technicians returned and released the mask, I had completed my first radiation treatment.

I had also learned how difficult the next seven weeks might become.

I wrote to Dr. Ricky and asked for something stronger to help me through the next few sessions. Even while asking, the old belief returned that I was inconveniencing everyone.

None of the doctors or technicians had treated me like a burden. The feeling came from somewhere much older than cancer. I had carried it since childhood, the belief that my needs interrupted other people's lives and that asking for help made me difficult.

That belief was no longer something I could afford to protect. I was fifty-six years old and had cancer. If there was ever a time to place my needs ahead of the fear of annoying someone, this was it.

After radiation, Kim and I went to a Persian restaurant. I wanted to eat while food still tasted normal and swallowing remained possible.

I ate too much and felt terrible afterward. I could not tell whether the discomfort came from the chemotherapy, the meal, or both, so I blamed the food because that seemed easier.

We stopped at Target for pillows and a thermometer. While walking through the store, I began feeling dizzy and wanted to leave as quickly as possible.

The first day had begun before sunrise and included hours of chemotherapy, radiation, walking between buildings, and the emotional strain of the mask. By the time we returned to the hotel, my body had reached its limit.

I called my parents and updated them. I also spoke with Joan, Kelley, my brother Mark, and Mark's wife, Ann Marie.

Talking to my family helped me feel like myself. I joked about the fact that the cancer was connected to HPV and ran some of the material past Mark and Ann Marie. The expression on my brother's face and my sister-in-law's laughter gave me a moment of normality.

Cancer had already taken control of my calendar, but it did not have to control every conversation.

My sponsor called later that night. He had been with me for nearly twenty years and understood the history behind every fear I had about medication.

I explained the treatments and the level of pain the doctors expected later. I told him I intended to remain as comfortable as possible and would take whatever was medically necessary.

He did not lecture me. He listened while I poured out everything that had accumulated during the day.

I told him how much his guidance had meant throughout my sobriety, including the things he had taught me without realizing he was teaching them. Recovery had given me the ability to live one day at a time, and that had never felt more important.

Seven weeks of treatment sounded impossible when I tried to experience all of it at once. One day was something I might be able to handle.

My concept of God had changed throughout recovery. I did not believe in a punishing God who had given me cancer because of something I had done. I believed there was something greater than me moving through people, circumstances, service, and the connections that appeared when I needed them.

The hands holding mine beneath the mask had felt like part of that.

The diagnosis had also strengthened my desire to make Ryan's Rockstars into something permanent. I imagined raising money through music, golf tournaments, auctions, and other events to create joyful experiences for children fighting cancer.

I also began imagining another organization that could connect cancer patients who were alone with survivors or volunteers willing to accompany them. I had no complete plan for it, but the purpose was clear. Nobody should have to face treatment alone unless that was what they chose.

I had received an extraordinary amount of support because my work placed me in front of people. Friends, family, performers, fans, neighbors, and members of my recovery community knew what I was facing.

Other patients did not have that visibility. Some entered treatment with no Donny, Chris, neighbors, patched performers, or parents calling to ask how they were doing.

My cancer had to become useful for them somehow. I did not yet know whether I would survive long enough to create any of those organizations, but imagining them gave the experience a purpose beyond my own body.

The next day, I had only one medical appointment scheduled. Radiation was not until 6:50 that evening.

I spoke with my oldest brother, Rick, and we talked about the type of cancer I had.

Rick had given me my first drumsticks when I was seven years old and helped start the musical life that eventually became my career. He and my other brothers had lived much more conventional-looking lives. They wore short hair, had no tattoos, and probably never expected their youngest brother to become the long-haired, heavily tattooed owner of a national entertainment company.

I had always considered myself the black sheep of the family. At fifty-six, none of those outward differences seemed important.

What mattered was seeing my brothers' faces and hearing their voices. I wished we lived closer, especially now that my parents were too old to travel easily.

At approximately six, Donny and I walked back to the radiation department. I had taken half a milligram of Ativan an hour before the appointment, but I did not feel any effect.

The department was running behind because of an emergency. When my turn came, two technicians I had not worked with the day before brought me into the room.

They were not unkind. They were moving quickly, speaking quickly, and attempting to get the treatment back on schedule.

That speed was enough to trigger me.

They positioned me, placed the bite guard in my mouth, and began securing the mask before I had found the small degree of comfort I needed.

Panic arrived immediately.

The pressure across my face and neck became connected to every failure I had ever experienced. Failed relationships, failed jobs, failed business decisions, addiction, shame, and the darkest parts of the pandemic rushed into the room at once.

Now I believed I was failing at cancer treatment too.

I had spent years imagining that cancer would eventually arrive, and during the pandemic, I often felt as though hands were closing around my throat. The mask recreated that sensation physically. I was locked down, my neck could not move, and my mind began telling me that I would not survive another minute.

The Ativan was doing almost nothing.

I could not understand why I was unable to tolerate the mask. Other people completed the same treatment every day. The technicians were trying to help me, and the machine was there to save my life.

None of those facts affected the panic.

I began kicking and signaling that I needed to be released. The technicians stopped and removed the mask.

I sat up crying. They told me I could take a break and reassured me that nothing I was doing was wrong.

Their kindness almost made me cry harder. They were doing everything possible to help, and I still could not control myself.

I walked out to the lobby where Donny was waiting. The expression on his face changed as soon as he saw me.

"I can't do it," I told him. "I can't fucking do it."

The tears became heavier. Trying to stop them only made the crying more violent.

I worried that crying would swell my throat and block my nose, making it even harder to complete the treatment. Every reaction created another reason to panic.

I went into the bathroom, washed my face, blew my nose, and took another Ativan. Other patients offered encouragement while they waited for their treatments.

They believed I was afraid of cancer or dying. I was not sure how to explain that the greatest fear was failure.

The mask opened doors inside my head that I could not organize. I did not understand why those memories were connected or why being physically restrained gave them so much power.

The other patients completed their appointments. I remained in the lobby while the medication had time to enter my system.

Eventually, I was the last person waiting.

The technicians brought me back into the room. One of the people who had helped me the previous day joined them. They told me to move slightly beneath the mask until I found the position that felt least uncomfortable.

They lowered it slowly and fastened it without rushing. I concentrated on breathing and tried not to think beyond the next few seconds.

This time, I completed the treatment.

Finishing did not make me feel victorious. I felt emotionally destroyed.

When they released me, I needed a hug. I did not know whether technicians were supposed to hug patients or whether some professional boundary prohibited it.

I asked anyway, and they gave me one.

Donny brought me back to the hotel. By then, the additional Ativan had finally begun working, and I fell asleep hard.

The next treatment was scheduled for 7:40 the following morning.

I woke feeling disoriented. The cause might have been the Ativan, chemotherapy, lack of sleep, or the cumulative stress of the previous two days.

My acid reflux was severe, but the appointment was approaching, so I took another Ativan. I had learned that waiting until I reached the treatment room was too late.

Donny and I arrived early, and the technicians offered to bring me in ahead of schedule. I declined because I wanted the medication to have every possible minute to work.

One of the technicians had witnessed the previous night's collapse. The staff moved more slowly this time, allowing me to settle onto the table before fastening the mask.

They cut small eyeholes into it. Being able to see a little of the room made the restraint feel less complete.

I requested The Beatles. Once the mask was secured, the technicians moved quickly out of the room so the treatment could begin.

Their voices came through the microphone. I heard the machine taking its positioning images and then the announcement that the radiation was starting.

"Oh! Darling" began playing.

It was one of the first Beatles songs I remembered learning and one of the most difficult songs to sing properly. Hearing it while unable to move my mouth created another strange connection between music and the body I was trying to preserve.

Postnasal drainage continued entering my throat. I swallowed because the alternative felt like choking, even though every swallow increased my fear of moving.

I made it through the procedure. I remained anxious, but the panic did not reach the level it had the previous night.

Before they released me, I insisted they take photographs of me wearing the mask. I wanted people to understand what head-and-neck radiation looked like.

From the outside, cancer treatment could be reduced to phrases such as "He's getting radiation" or "She's doing chemotherapy." The words did not show the table, the bite guard, the pressure across the face, or the moment when everyone left the room.

The photographs would.

As soon as the mask came off, another form of panic arrived. I had completed the treatment, but I already knew I would have to return after the holiday weekend and do it again.

Support surrounded me. Donny was nearby, my family was calling, and the staff had shown extraordinary patience.

The reality remained that once the mask was secured and the technicians left, I was alone on the table.

I needed every ounce of human contact I could receive during that period. The handshakes and hugs were not small gestures. They reminded my body that I had not been abandoned.

Later that morning, I attended my first appointment with the palliative-care team. I understood palliative care as comfort care, the people responsible for helping manage pain, anxiety, nausea, and the other symptoms created by treatment.

A nurse and social worker met with me. Their approach was soft and unhurried. They let me speak in my own language, including the profanity, fear, and frustration.

I told them that I did not know which questions I was supposed to ask. I knew only that I did not want to be in unnecessary pain.

We discussed the anxiety caused by the mask, the nausea and reflux after chemotherapy, and the increasing pain in my right hand. I had not attempted to hold a guitar pick since my final show.

They talked about medication, support groups, and other forms of assistance. I was willing to consider whatever they believed would help.

The subject of medical cannabis came up again. Friends, family members, people in recovery, and cancer survivors had all suggested gummies for nausea, appetite, sleep, pain, and anxiety.

For most patients, that decision might not have carried much emotional weight. For me, it crossed a boundary I had protected for nearly twenty years.

For two decades, survival meant staying away from intoxicating substances. Marijuana had been part of the life I left behind, and my sobriety date represented every day since I had stopped using.

Now people were suggesting that one of those substances might help me survive cancer.

My sponsor and longtime friends in recovery did not object. They understood the difference between seeking intoxication and treating symptoms created by chemotherapy and radiation.

A friend from high school whom I had not spoken with in decades owned several cannabis shops and had offered to help. During the drive back to Visalia, I contacted him and asked about gummies for pain, nausea, reflux, and anxiety.

I told him to charge me whatever they cost. He said he would arrange it.

The decision still made me uncomfortable. Sobriety had become part of how I understood myself, and I did not want anyone to believe I had used cancer as an excuse to get high.

That fear of judgment revealed how much power I still gave other people's opinions. None of them were beneath the mask with me, feeling the nausea, or attempting to swallow through a throat being damaged by radiation.

This was not about protecting an image. It was about staying alive.

When I returned home that weekend, Smokey meowed for approximately forty-five minutes. He followed me through the house as though he needed to account for every hour I had been away.

My body was exhausted. I drank some water, ate a little, rinsed my mouth with the solutions the hospital had recommended, and returned to bed.

When I woke in the afternoon, Donny was standing above me. He had come to say goodbye before leaving for a performance.

I had nearly forgotten that it was Saturday.

Four Killer Dueling Pianos teams were performing that night. Donny and Chris had a birthday event in Tulare. John and TJ were at La Jolla

Country Club. Nathan and Jason had a show in San Diego, while Steve, Johnny, and Mimi were performing at another San Diego birthday party.

Each team checked in and sent photographs of its setup. I sat at home recovering from chemotherapy while the company operated in four locations without me.

I called them my players, but the word never fully described the relationship. They were my brothers and sisters, and I was only the person trying to keep the ship moving in the right direction.

The fact that the company continued without me produced both pride and fear. I had built the systems and relationships necessary for it to operate, but surrendering control remained difficult.

Cancer was forcing me to trust the people I had said I trusted.

My energy and appetite improved later that day. I went to the country club and managed to eat four tacos and a bowl of ice cream.

Food still tasted normal enough to enjoy. The doctors had warned that this would change, but warnings remained theoretical until the changes actually arrived.

That evening, I spent time with Chris, Jenna, and their daughters. A mariachi band played somewhere in the neighborhood, possibly for a graduation, birthday, or quinceañera.

The drumming reminded me of marching band and my school friend, Mike Fisher, who had recently passed from cancer. Music continued pulling the living and dead into the same moment.

Before going to sleep, I noticed soreness developing on the right side of my throat. I used the baking-soda rinse and MuGard the hospital had given me.

The treatment had begun leaving its first visible marks.

The following day, I called my parents and discussed medical cannabis. I expected the conversation to be uncomfortable because they had spent twenty years being proud of my sobriety.

Instead, my mother told me to give myself a break. My father said the only thing that mattered was saving my life.

I began crying while speaking with them. Their response told me that using a medication during and post cancer treatment would not change how they saw me or erase the work I had done.

I had always known my parents loved me. In that conversation, I felt closer to them than I had in a long time.

I also called Kimber Breaux while driving back toward UCLA. She had approximately seventeen more years of sobriety than I did and had been a guiding presence since our time together in the Bummkinn Band.

Her father had died around the time I received the diagnosis, so I had hesitated to place my problems on top of her grief. When I finally asked about cannabis, she gave the same answer as everyone else.

This was cancer. This was treatment. It did not change my sobriety date.

Sobriety existed to save lives, and in that moment, the life we were attempting to save was mine.

Radiation continued on May 26 and May 27. I still needed Ativan before the mask went on.

Donny returned the night before my second chemotherapy session because he wanted to make sure I reached the seven o'clock appointment. He continued trying to balance the company, performances, his personal responsibilities, and my care.

I worried about the amount of pressure he was carrying. He rarely complained, which did not mean the weight was not there.

The second chemotherapy session began early on May 28. I told the nurse about the nausea and acid reflux I had experienced after the first infusion.

She contacted the doctor and added medication for the reflux to my IV. The difference was significant, and I did not experience the same burning discomfort afterward.

Dr. Deborah visited during the infusion. Like the rest of the UCLA team, she wanted to know what could be adjusted to make treatment more tolerable.

I had entered cancer care expecting to be treated like a diagnosis. The people at UCLA kept treating me like a person.

After chemotherapy, I felt hungry and asked Donny to take me to a cannabis store. I wanted to understand what was available rather than continue discussing it as an abstract possibility.

The shop was nearly empty. A woman behind the counter explained different options and sold me gummies in two strengths, along with a concentrated cannabis oil.

Back at the hotel, Donny and I joked about which stereotypical stoner music I should play. Just as I opened the package, my sponsor called.

The timing created another round of laughter. Nobody involved treated the moment as a relapse or moral crisis. We were trying to find something that might reduce symptoms and help me eat.

I took one of the lower-dose gummies and a small amount of the oil.

Nothing happened.

There was no meaningful relief and no noticeable intoxication. I remembered that the first time I tried marijuana as a teenager, I did not feel anything either.

The experience was almost anticlimactic after the emotional struggle required to permit it.

The next day, Donny had to leave for work. Johnny joined him for a performance in Paso Robles, while Steve and another player handled a show in Bakersfield.

I had three medical appointments and faced the day largely on my own.

The first was an IV infusion for hydration. I had been advised to receive additional fluids throughout treatment, and I liked the appointments because I usually felt better afterward.

The next appointment was a hearing test. So far, the results did not show a noticeable change from my baseline.

That evening, I took half an Ativan before radiation. A team I had not worked with previously handled the treatment. They did their best, and I completed it.

When I returned to the hotel, I tried one of the stronger gummies.

Approximately an hour and a half later, I felt the effects. The nausea disappeared, my appetite returned, and I ate almost everything available in the room.

The gummy had done exactly what people said it might do.

I did not particularly enjoy being stoned, though.

After twenty years of mental clarity, the altered feeling was no longer comforting. The younger version of me had sought that separation from reality. The sober version wanted relief without losing control of his mind.

That distinction mattered. The substance was helping certain symptoms, but I did not want the experience itself.

The following morning, radiation was scheduled at ten. I intended to drive back to Visalia afterward, so taking any sedating substance beforehand was not an option.

I arrived anxious but relieved to see technicians I recognized. The familiar team understood the routine that had developed around my hair, the mask, and the time I needed before they left the room.

The treatment remained uncomfortable. Postnasal drainage continued triggering the need to swallow even though the mask restricted the movement.

They played The Beatles, and I made it through.

Afterward, I met with Dr. Ricky and his nurse practitioner, Jasmine. I had begun calling the radiation treatments Dr. Ricky's Nuclear Barbecue.

Both of them approached my progress with optimism. They said everything appeared to be lining up properly and gave me more lotion for the skin around my face and neck.

They also reminded me that I was still in the early portion of treatment. The fact that I was not yet experiencing severe pain did not mean it would remain that way.

On the way back to the hotel, three inquiries for shows came through. I could have waited until I reached Visalia, but years of running the company had taught me that ten minutes could be the difference between booking a client and losing one.

I returned the calls, sent quotes, packed the room, and drove home.

By the time I reached Visalia, nausea had returned. I took another gummy, which removed the nausea and made it possible to eat.

Once again, I disliked the feeling of being high.

Donny and Johnny were performing locally that night. When they returned to the house, I was asleep on the couch.

I was grateful they were there. The cats stayed close, as though they recognized that the battle had moved into another stage.

The following morning, May 31, I woke with the first throat pain I would describe as severe. My appetite was gone.

Four contract requests were waiting. Each contract normally took only several minutes to prepare, but focusing on them required nearly everything I had.

The company did not stop because my throat hurt. Clients still wanted answers, and performers still needed the work.

I forced myself to finish the documents while the temperature outside reached approximately 105 degrees.

I had been dictating my daily events since my diagnosis, but now the diary had been paused for a week.

The silence was not caused by a lack of events. I no longer had the energy to record them.

Fighting cancer had become a full-time job. Appointments, medication, rinses, food, hydration, travel, radiation, chemotherapy, and pain occupied nearly every part of the day.

The throat pain intensified until every swallow felt as though razor blades were moving through me. Drinking hurt. Eating hurt. Blowing my nose hurt.

The morphine I had been prescribed did not provide enough relief.

Radiation was damaging the inside of my mouth and throat. Blisters formed, burst, and returned. Food that had been tolerable one day could cause an immediate explosion of pain the next.

Kelley Patrick arrived from Ohio during the first week of June. We had known each other for approximately thirty-five years, and she was one of my closest friends.

She also understood cats, which mattered almost as much as anything else. She could help care for Sophie, Meg, and Smokey while I traveled between Visalia and UCLA.

Having her there was generous and loving. I was also becoming emotionally toxic.

Pain made me sensitive to every question, movement, and attempt at conversation. I did not want anyone too close, even though I was terrified of being alone.

That contradiction was difficult for both of us. I needed help but resented the vulnerability that made help necessary.

I was fighting more than cancer. The treatments had reopened fear, shame, addiction memories, pandemic trauma, and the belief that I was an undeserving burden.

Kelley could not solve any of that. She could only remain nearby, care for the cats, and help with practical things while I became increasingly difficult to reach.

After radiation on Friday, we returned to Visalia. Steve and Johnny were also in the Central Valley for a wedding, and Kim had left potato soup in the refrigerator.

The soup tasted good for the brief moment I could taste it. Almost immediately, the inside of my mouth erupted in blisters.

The radiation seemed to be peeling away the tissue inside my mouth and throat.

Then I discovered that I could no longer yawn properly.

A yawn is something most people never consider. The mouth opens, the throat expands, the breath enters, and the movement reaches a natural release.

My body still initiated the yawn, but the burned tissue could not complete the motion.

The pressure built inside my jaw and throat while I attempted to open my mouth. Pain stopped the movement before it could finish, leaving me trapped in the middle.

I howled, huffed, and struggled to breathe through it. The more I tried to force the yawn, the more anxiety tightened my body.

The experience sounds almost ridiculous when described aloud. I could not yawn.

Inside my body, it felt like torture.

The unfinished movement created panic unlike anything I expected from radiation. The only comparison I could produce for swallowing was trying to force down a pine cone.

I managed some noodles and protein shakes. Every attempt to consume something required concentration and willingness to accept pain.

Payroll still had to be completed. The performers were out working, and I had to make sure they were paid.

I wanted only to hold the cats and sleep.

By June 9, the condition of my mouth had improved slightly because some of the blisters had burst. The relief was temporary.

I decided Kelley should remain in Visalia with the cats while I drove back to UCLA. I arrived around one in the afternoon with enough energy to believe the day might be manageable.

Then another yawn began.

I sat in the hotel room attempting to complete it. The movement stopped halfway, and panic rushed through me.

The walls seemed to close in. I could not breathe properly, could not release the pressure in my throat, and could not convince my body that an unfinished yawn was not going to kill me.

I went to the hospital early and walked into the palliative-care department without an appointment.

Kristin, one of the nurses, came out to speak with me. The moment I attempted to explain what was happening, I began crying.

I hated crying in front of people. It made me feel exposed and out of control.

I told her that I could not complete a yawn and understood how absurd that sounded. The problem was not the word. It was the pain, pressure, panic, and inability to escape my own throat.

I wanted the pain to stop. I wanted my mind shut down.

Kristin sat with me and listened. The team planned to try gabapentin, a medication I had not been seeking.

I wanted a strong cough syrup I had previously used when a sore throat threatened a singing performance. I knew that medication had provided relief in the past and wanted something familiar.

Cancer treatment did not operate according to what had helped me perform years earlier. I had to try what the medical team believed was appropriate.

I also had a hydration infusion scheduled nearby. When I sat in the chair, the nurse attempted to place the IV.

I began sobbing again.

Whether I was dehydrated, panicking, or simply had veins exhausted by repeated needles, the IV would not go in easily. The nurses tried several times before finding a usable vein.

I knew they were skilled and doing everything possible to help. The failed attempts were not anyone's fault.

Each needle intensified the feeling that my body was no longer cooperating with anything.

The tears would not stop. Nurses gathered around me while the fluids finally began entering the vein.

I told them I wanted to be blacked out for the remainder of treatment. I did not want mild medication, breathing exercises, or encouragement.

My history with opiates meant I knew what strong medication could do. I knew the feeling of pain receding and the mind becoming quiet.

I was not asking because I wanted to return to addiction. I was asking because I did not want to experience another minute of what was happening.

A full panic attack took over. I could not breathe properly, could not finish the yawn, and could not stop crying.

The situation pulled me back into the emotional experience of the pandemic. I felt trapped, isolated, furious, and unable to escape a world that had closed around me.

The medical team tried to guide my breathing. They contacted the nurse practitioner and added lorazepam to the IV.

Gradually, the panic loosened enough for me to think.

What remained was darkness.

I no longer wanted to tell people what I was going through. Every time I opened up, someone offered advice, encouragement, or another reason I was supposed to feel hopeful.

I did not want another person telling me I was brave.

I did not feel brave. I felt trapped inside treatment that was destroying the tissue in my throat so that it could destroy the cancer.

The staff mentioned psychological support. I resisted the idea because I did not want anyone treating my reaction as though it meant I was dangerous to myself or others.

I did not intend to harm anyone, including myself. I wanted relief.

There was a difference.

My brother Sean called while I was still connected to the IV. I told him what had happened and admitted that I no longer cared whether I lived or died.

That did not mean I planned to end my life. It meant the fight had lost its emotional meaning.

The following morning, I had another swallowing-preservation appointment. We did not spend much time discussing exercises.

I told the clinician about the previous day, the panic, the IV attempts, and the sense that the medications were not controlling the pain. I believed everyone was pussyfooting around the problem, giving me small amounts of medication while my mouth and throat were being burned away.

I wanted something strong enough to do the job.

She listened without diminishing what I described. She reminded me that the treatment was extremely difficult and that I did not need to minimize it simply because other patients had worse diagnoses.

That was difficult for me to accept.

My cancer had strong survival odds compared with many others. Friends of mine were facing diseases their doctors could not cure, while I was receiving treatment people expected to work.

I felt ungrateful for collapsing under something I had been told I would likely survive.

At the same time, statistics no longer comforted me. Nearly everyone had originally believed the mass in my neck was probably not cancer.

The favorable odds had been wrong then. I did not know why I should surrender my fear to another percentage now.

I did not want motivational slogans from friends or family. I did not want to be told how strong I was by people who were not lying beneath the mask or trying to swallow with the inside of their throat burned.

I was not even certain I would have listened to someone who had experienced the same treatment. Every body, mind, and cancer journey was different.

My spiritual connection also felt absent. I still believed God existed, but belief did not create comfort.

God's will would be done whether I approved of it or not. If heaven was real and death brought peace, I could not understand why everyone insisted that remaining alive through unbearable treatment was automatically the better outcome.

Or was everything I had ever been told about God and Heaven a lie?

I guess I have a different God.

I questioned whether I was extending life or extending misery.

The optimism I carried into the first treatment had disappeared. The cancer warrior language no longer fit what I felt.

I did not want to inspire anyone. I wanted to be numb.

Chemotherapy and radiation continued. The appointments remained on the calendar, and the mask was still waiting for me each weekday.

The treatments had not stopped, but my ability to carry them independently was disappearing.

I had begun the process believing I could work from the chemotherapy chair, manage contracts from the hotel, return home on weekends, and keep enough control over my life to remain recognizable to myself.

Three weeks later, eating had become a battle, swallowing felt like razor blades, morphine was not controlling the pain, and a yawn could send me into a full panic attack.

The hotel room was still close to the hospital, but close was no longer enough. I needed more than appointments, prescriptions, and occasional hydration.

I needed the kind of care that could not be carried back to Room 152 in a paper bag.

CHAPTER FIFTEEN

No Bell

"There be no more ahhhhhhhhh!"

SONG: COMFORTABLY NUMB
BAND: PINK FLOYD

By the middle of June, I could no longer pretend that I was capable of managing the treatment from a hotel room. The pain had moved beyond something I could work around, and the medication I had been taking outside the hospital was not controlling it.

Every swallow felt like fire. The tissue inside my mouth and throat had been burned, blistered, and stripped by weeks of radiation. Drinking water hurt, but not drinking created dehydration, which made everything else worse. Food was no longer something I enjoyed or even tolerated. It had become a physical test I repeatedly failed.

I had begun treatment believing I could organize my way through it. I had reserved the Tiverton for seven weeks, packed the right foods, arranged help for the cats, prepared the performers, and carried my laptop to appointments. I imagined returning to the hotel after radiation, answering calls, completing contracts, and driving home on weekends.

That plan belonged to a body I no longer had.

Kelley's time in California was nearing its end. She had done everything she could, including caring for Sophie, Meg, and Smokey while I traveled between Visalia and UCLA. I had been difficult to help because pain had made me angry, withdrawn, and sensitive to almost every attempt at conversation.

I needed her presence, but I also wanted everyone to leave me alone. There was no reasonable way for another person to satisfy both of those needs.

Around the middle of June, on what I remember as a Sunday, the pain became impossible to manage. The doctors and nurses had repeatedly told me that if it became severe, I should go to the emergency room.

I finally went.

The emergency-room staff gave me an injection of Dilaudid. The relief was almost immediate. The fire in my throat receded, my body relaxed, and for the first time in days, I was no longer focused entirely on pain.

I had spent weeks asking for that level of relief. The experience confirmed what I had been trying to explain: the pain could be controlled if the medication was strong enough.

The Dilaudid did not solve the underlying problem. It gave me a temporary break from it.

I returned to the hotel believing I might be able to rest. By that evening, the medication had worn off, and the pain came back harder.

I could no longer remain in the room. Kelley was there, but I told her to stay behind while I attempted to return to the emergency department.

I tried to order a ride. None arrived.

The hospital was only a few blocks away, which normally would not have seemed significant. Under treatment, with my throat on fire and my body weakened by chemotherapy, radiation, dehydration, and lack of food, the distance felt much greater.

I walked.

Every step increased my anger. I had spent years crossing airports, carrying equipment, loading trucks, climbing stairs, and performing for hours. Now three blocks between a hotel and a hospital felt like a test of whether I could remain upright.

When I reached the emergency department, the waiting area was crowded. Several family members had accompanied one patient and occupied most of the available seating.

I was in agony and could not find a chair.

Eventually, I sat outside on the ground.

The humiliation of that moment stayed with me. I was a cancer patient in severe pain, sitting in the dirt outside an emergency room because nobody inside seemed willing to move so I could have a chair.

I understood that the people in the waiting area were frightened about someone they loved. I also understood that fear did not remove the need for basic awareness of the people around you.

I did not need seven family members explaining my symptoms, offering opinions, or competing with one another over what should happen next. I needed one person beside me and a chair.

The hospital staff brought me water, but swallowing it was almost impossible. I remained outside for what felt like hours, shifting positions because no position made the pain tolerable.

Eventually, I was moved into a temporary area inside a tent. From there, they brought me into the emergency department.

By then, Chris knew I had returned. I had also been communicating with Kelley and Donny, although the details of those conversations became less clear as the medication increased.

The hospital decided to admit me.

I had cancer, but cancer itself was not the official reason I remained in the hospital. I was admitted for palliative care because I could no longer control the pain or feed myself.

That distinction sounded strange at first. The cancer had created the treatment, and the treatment had created the condition that brought me into the emergency department. Still, the immediate medical problem was comfort, hydration, nutrition, and the fact that my body could no longer manage outside the hospital.

There was not an ordinary inpatient room available immediately. I was placed in a small office-like area near the emergency department with a hospital chair that could extend into something resembling a bed.

It was not comfortable, but I had reached the point where the type of room did not matter. I wanted medication strong enough to stop the pain.

Kelley wanted to remain in Los Angeles and postpone her flight home. She had traveled across the country to help me and did not want to leave while I was being admitted.

I told her to go.

She had already given me more than I had known how to receive. I also knew that Alex was traveling to California and would arrive soon. Alex was an ex-girlfriend, a nurse, a cancer survivor, and someone I had known since our years in Columbus.

Kelley cried, and I understood why. Leaving somebody in a hospital feels wrong, especially when you do not know how long he will remain there or whether his condition will improve.

I could not ask her to abandon the rest of her life indefinitely. I told her that I would be surrounded by medical staff and other friends.

Eventually, she left for the airport.

I remained in the emergency area for approximately a day and a half, although my memory of the timeline became unreliable. Medication, exhaustion, dehydration, and pain blurred the hours together.

At some point, the hospital moved me into an inpatient room. I do not clearly remember the transfer.

By then, the doctors were finally giving me medication strong enough to produce meaningful relief. I had spent weeks trying to remain coherent while my throat burned. Now coherence became less important than comfort.

The palliative-care team placed me on a patient-controlled morphine pump. The device allowed me to press a button and receive a measured dose when the pain increased.

The machine prevented me from giving myself more than the doctors considered safe. If I pressed the button too soon, it simply would not deliver another dose.

For the first time, I had some control over when relief arrived.

The medication entered, created a powerful rush of calm, and often allowed me to fall asleep for a while. I did not have to call a nurse and wait until someone became available each time the pain surged.

I could press the button.

The history behind that action was not lost on me. Twenty years earlier, I had nearly destroyed my life chasing the exact feeling strong narcotics could provide. Now a hospital had placed the relief in my hand and told me to use it when needed.

The difference was context, intention, and medical supervision. I was not using drugs to escape an ordinary life. I was using them because the inside of my throat had been burned by the treatment intended to keep me alive.

Still, my body recognized the feeling.

The relief could become almost blissful for a few moments. Pain disappeared, anxiety loosened, and the noise inside my mind became quieter. After weeks of fighting for every swallow, those moments felt enormous.

When the palliative-care physician came to evaluate me, I explained that the strongest relief occurred when the medication created that initial rush and allowed me to drift out of consciousness.

I told him that I believed that effect needed to remain part of the treatment. I did not want the medication adjusted so lightly that I stayed awake and miserable simply because everyone was afraid of making me too comfortable.

He listened and agreed.

The doctors began giving me regular pain medication and anxiety medication in addition to the doses available through the pump. I became far more comfortable than I had been in the hotel.

Comfort did not mean I was well. It meant I was no longer fully present for every minute of suffering.

Alex arrived in Los Angeles shortly after I was admitted. We had dated during the 1990s, and I had once written and recorded a song about her. Our lives had moved in different directions, but the friendship remained.

Her being a nurse gave me a level of reassurance that another visitor might not have provided. She understood hospitals, medications, alarms, medical conversations, and the condition of a patient who could move between clarity and confusion within minutes.

She had also survived cancer herself. She did not need me to explain that treatment could become more frightening than the disease.

Alex stayed in the Tiverton room I had reserved, but she spent much of her time at the hospital. I was often too medicated to carry a complete conversation, yet knowing she was there made the room feel less empty.

Steve Weatherby also came to see me. Steve and I had lived together near the Ohio State campus, and our bands had shared stages in Columbus. I had not seen him in approximately fifteen years.

That evening, he and Alex sat near the foot of the hospital bed talking while I drifted in and out of awareness. I remember trying to participate, pressing the morphine button, and then disappearing into sleep again.

The scene felt like different parts of my past had entered the same room. Alex and Steve belonged to a younger version of me, the musician who was still drinking, using pills, chasing bands, and believing he had unlimited time.

Now they were sitting beside a hospital bed while that same body was being treated for cancer.

I could not remain awake long enough to understand what their presence meant. I knew only that they had come.

Even with the improved pain control, I still could not eat. The radiation had damaged my mouth and throat so severely that swallowing enough calories was no longer realistic.

My body needed nutrition if I was going to complete treatment. The doctors decided to place a feeding tube directly into my stomach.

I had attended swallowing-preservation appointments and completed exercises partly because I wanted to avoid this outcome. The feeding tube had been presented as a possibility, not something I expected to need.

By the time the doctors recommended it, I had no meaningful argument left. I was losing weight, unable to consume enough calories, and dependent on IV fluids.

The tube was no longer an inconvenience. It had become the available way to keep my body functioning.

A few days into the hospital stay, they prepared to take me to the operating room. My throat was unbearably dry because I was not allowed to drink before the procedure.

I kept asking for water.

The residents told me they were going to put me under soon and that I needed to wait. One doctor eventually brought me a wet cloth that I could place in my mouth and suck on.

The moisture was minimal, but even that small relief mattered.

I lay in the operating room looking at unfamiliar faces and waiting for the anesthesia. Then someone I recognized walked toward me wearing hospital scrubs and a gown.

It was Chris.

He had seen my name on the surgical schedule and came to check on me. He was not the anesthesiologist assigned to the procedure, but he was working that day and had noticed that I was there.

For a moment, the operating room stopped feeling completely foreign. I had known Chris since we were teenagers playing music in Ohio. He was the person who had helped get me into UCLA, guided me through the appointments, and translated parts of the medical system when I could not understand them.

Now he was standing beside me moments before another procedure.

"What the fuck are you doing here?" I asked.

I also told him to find me some water.

The humor was imperfect because I was desperate, but it was still humor. Seeing Chris allowed that part of me to return briefly.

Then the anesthesia took over.

When I woke, the feeding tube extended from my abdomen. The hospital staff began teaching me how nutrition would enter my body without passing through my mouth.

The process was physically simple compared with eating. Formula could travel through the tube and reach my stomach without touching the burned tissue in my throat.

Emotionally, it was another loss of independence.

Eating is connected to almost everything. It is nourishment, routine, pleasure, celebration, travel, family, and social life. I had joined the country club partly because I wanted good meals when I returned from the road. Now food could enter my body while I tasted nothing and swallowed nothing.

The tube kept me alive, but it also confirmed how far treatment had taken me from ordinary life.

Hospitalization did not interrupt radiation. The staff placed me in a wheelchair and transported me through the hospital to the radiation department five days a week.

The route became part of my routine. Instead of walking from the Tiverton, I left the inpatient floor with hospital identification around my wrist, medication in my body, and a tube entering my stomach.

The technicians already knew me. They had seen the early panic, the failed attempts, the tears, and the days when getting the mask over my face seemed nearly impossible.

By then, I was receiving stronger pain and anxiety medication, and my relationship with the mask had changed. It was still restrictive, but it no longer produced the same immediate terror every time.

Part of the change came from medication. Part came from repetition, and part came from the fact that I had already survived so many sessions.

The mask was no longer an unknown threat. It was a miserable procedure with a beginning and an end.

Chemotherapy also continued from the hospital when my blood counts permitted it. Rather than requiring me to report to the outpatient infusion center, the drugs could be brought to the room or administered while I was already under inpatient care.

Cancer treatment continued whether I felt prepared for it or not. Being admitted did not pause the schedule. It changed the location from which I endured it.

The hospital bed became the center of my life. I received medications, nutrition, blood tests, consultations, and business calls from the same place.

Somehow, I continued operating The Killer Dueling Pianos.

Clients called without knowing I was connected to tubes. Emails arrived, contracts needed to be prepared, and payroll still had to be processed. I answered when I was coherent enough and returned to sleep when the medication took over.

The laptop rested near the bed. I typed contracts from a hospital room and spoke to clients while attempting to sound as though everything was under control.

Part of that was dedication. Part of it was my inability to release control completely.

The company had extraordinary people carrying it. Donny, Johnny, Steve, Jami, John, and the other performers handled the events and made decisions without pulling me into every problem.

They checked in, visited when possible, and continued protecting the reputation of the company. Nobody used my illness as a reason to lower the standard.

I had spent years telling people that the patch represented family. Cancer proved whether that statement was real.

They did not merely send messages saying they hoped I felt better. They worked, covered the dates, communicated with clients, and allowed me to remain a patient without fearing that everything I had built would collapse.

Donny carried more than anyone should have been expected to carry. He continued performing, managing parts of the company, visiting me, checking on the house, and making sure the cats were cared for.

There was no job description for what he was doing. Brotherhood was the only explanation.

Even from the hospital bed, I continued receiving financial and administrative problems. The IRS eventually returned the eleven thousand dollars I had paid while disputing their claim.

Getting my own money back cost approximately twenty-eight hundred dollars in professional fees. That seemed perfectly consistent with the logic of the situation: the government had made the mistake, I had paid to prevent further trouble, and I then had to pay someone else to recover the money.

The refund check was sent to my house. Donny placed it safely in a drawer, and I forgot about it for weeks.

Before cancer, eleven thousand dollars would have received my immediate attention. In the hospital, it became a piece of paper in a drawer.

The meaning of money had changed again.

During the day, people often visited or called. Medical staff entered regularly, and appointments created movement around me. The activity helped prevent the room from feeling completely isolated.

The nights were different.

At night, the visitors left, the hallways became quieter, and the distance from my family felt larger. My parents were too old to travel across the country, and my brothers had responsibilities that made immediate visits difficult.

They called, FaceTimed, and supported me from wherever they were. I never doubted their love.

Love through a screen did not replace the presence of someone sitting beside the bed at two in the morning.

There were nights when I woke screaming because the medication had worn off. Pain could return before I was fully conscious, and the first thing I understood was that my throat was on fire.

I hit the call button and begged someone to come.

The night nurses were extraordinary. They entered without judgment, spoke calmly, and acted as though relieving my fear was as important as administering the medication.

One male nurse had a way of repeating that he had me.

"I've got you, buddy," he would say. "You're going to be okay. I've got you."

Then he would administer the medication through the line, and relief would begin moving through me.

The pain receded, anxiety loosened, and I could sleep again.

Those moments remain difficult to remember. There was comfort when the medication arrived, but there was also a level of loneliness I cannot fully describe.

Cancer had surrounded me with more support than many people ever receive, yet the most frightening nights still belonged to me alone. Nobody else could inhabit the body experiencing the burns, the feeding tube, the mask, or the fear that treatment might fail.

People can stand beside someone who is dying, but they cannot die for him. The same was true of treatment. People could drive me, feed the cats, take over the company, comb my hair, and hold my hand.

I still had to occupy the body.

Alex remained in town for approximately a week. During that time, I had not taken a proper shower. The staff had helped clean me in bed, but my long hair had become tangled and knotted.

Donny bought detangler and a brush. Alex sat beside me and slowly worked through the knots until my hair could be washed.

There was something deeply tender about the process. I had dated Alex when both of us were young, physically independent, and moving through the Columbus music scene. Now she was carefully pulling knots out of my hair because I could not manage it myself.

Taking a shower created another kind of vulnerability. I was weak enough that someone needed to remain nearby in case I became dizzy or fell.

I was also uncomfortable undressing in front of Alex. We had dated decades earlier, but that history did not remove the humiliation of being physically dependent.

She seemed to recognize the discomfort. Without making a speech, she removed the formality from the situation in the most direct way possible, using the bathroom and urinating in front of me as though there were nothing unusual about either of us being there.

The message was clear: stop worrying about dignity and get into the shower.

In the strangest possible way, it was one of the kindest things she could have done. She made the situation ordinary enough that I could move through it.

I showered, washed my hair, and felt cleaner than I had in days. The act was physically exhausting, but it restored a small part of my humanity.

Cancer had reduced many accomplishments to things I once completed without thought. Taking a shower, standing for several minutes, or walking through the hallway could feel as significant as finishing a performance.

Alex eventually had to return to Ohio. Her leaving created another empty space in the room, but her presence had carried me through one of the most vulnerable parts of the hospital stay.

By the beginning of July, my oldest brother, Rick, came to Los Angeles.

He arrived carrying a teddy bear.

I could not have Sophie, Meg, or Smokey in the hospital, so the bear stayed beside me as a substitute for the comfort I normally received from them.

The moment Rick entered the room, I began crying.

I had spoken with my family repeatedly, but he was the first blood relative able to stand beside my hospital bed. The emotion came out before I could control it.

Rick was my oldest brother and had given me my first pair of drumsticks when I was seven years old. That gift began a musical journey neither of us could have predicted.

Now he was entering a room where music, family, illness, and the fear of death had all come together.

We listened to old songs and talked about music. When I had enough strength, he walked with me around the hospital complex.

Those moments were simple, which was exactly what I needed. He did not have to solve the cancer or tell me how to feel. He was my brother, and he was there.

Rick did not feel completely well during the visit. At around the same time, my blood counts dropped to a dangerous level.

The medical team stopped chemotherapy for approximately a week. My body had reached a point where continuing the drug on schedule carried too much risk.

Hearing that the blood counts were dangerously low frightened me, even though I was already inside a hospital. The treatment intended to save me could also reduce my body's ability to protect itself.

I was not in intensive care, but the situation was serious enough that chemotherapy had to wait.

Rick visited for two days. After returning to his hotel on the second night, he tested positive for COVID.

He changed his plans and prepared to return home.

I told the hospital staff that I had been exposed. Their response was far calmer than I expected after everything the world had experienced in 2020.

Nobody panicked. There was no dramatic lockdown of the room or immediate change in the treatment plan. Some staff wore masks, while others continued following whatever precautions they had already been using.

Several days later, the hospital tested me. The result was negative.

The contrast with the pandemic years was difficult not to notice. In 2020, the possibility of infection had shut down the company and changed the course of my personal life. In 2025, I was an immunocompromised cancer patient whose brother had tested positive after visiting, and the hospital treated it as a manageable medical concern.

I did not know what conclusion to draw from that. I was too sick to spend much energy arguing with the past.

Rick went home, and I remained in the hospital.

By then, my body looked and felt completely different. I had lost significant weight. My neck was darkened and burned from radiation, and the inside of my mouth remained filled with sores.

Nutrition entered through the feeding tube. Blood was drawn repeatedly, sometimes several times a day. Every result seemed capable of changing whether I received chemotherapy, another medication, or an additional day in the hospital.

The treatment calendar continued moving toward its end.

During that period, H, who was the last girlfriend I had in Baltimore before I left, contacted me. I was not sober yet when we broke up. We had not seen one another in approximately twenty years.

We had exchanged occasional messages, but the cancer brought us into more regular conversation. She told me she had been thinking about me and wanted to visit.

H represented another unfinished part of my past. When we were together, I had still been drinking every day, taking pills, and behaving like a terrible boyfriend. She had been right to leave.

I had changed since then, but the insecurity created by Red's departure remained. Part of me wanted to know that someone who entered my life could tolerate seeing me at my worst.

There was no more complete version of my worst than the person in that hospital bed. I was thin, medicated, frightened, dependent upon a feeding tube, and unsure whether treatment would work.

H's interest gave me another reason to imagine leaving the hospital. I began looking toward the possibility of seeing her after I returned home.

Hope does not always arrive in a pure or sensible form. Sometimes it is connected to an old relationship, a future show, a cat waiting at home, or a conversation you do not yet understand.

At that moment, the possibility of her visit helped me look beyond the hospital room.

The radiation treatments continued each weekday. Over time, I became more comfortable with the process that had nearly broken me during the first week.

The mask had not become pleasant. It still pinned my shoulders, neck, and head to the table, and swallowing remained difficult.

What changed was my relationship with the fear.

I no longer needed the same preparation before every session. The medical staff knew how to position me, and I knew the sequence of sounds the machine would make.

I had survived each previous treatment. Repetition transformed the unknown into something familiar enough to endure.

By the final sessions, I could enter the radiation room with a very different attitude from the one I carried on the second day.

Instead of telling the technicians that I could not do it, I walked in ready to begin.

"Let's fucking go," I told them.

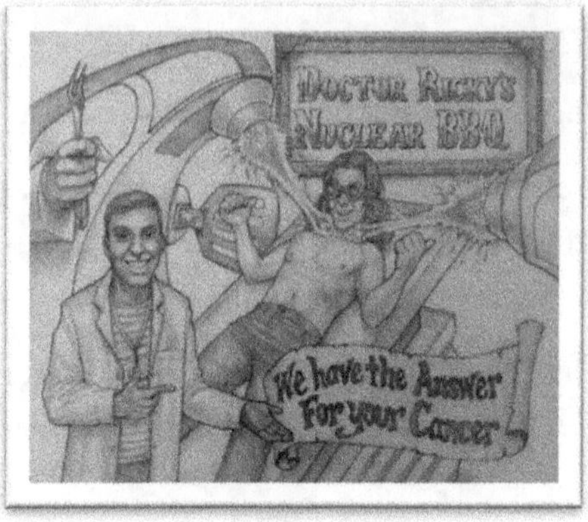

The confidence did not mean I was physically stronger. I was heavily medicated, underweight, burned, and being fed through a tube.

It meant the mask no longer owned my mind.

My voice also remained. It was rough, but it had not disappeared. Dr. Ricky's confidence that the radiation could avoid my vocal cords had proved justified so far.

I had spent the entire treatment fearing that cancer might take the one instrument I had carried since childhood. Hearing myself speak, even from a damaged throat, felt like evidence that part of me had survived.

Throughout treatment, I had referred to the radiation as Dr. Ricky's Barbecue. As the end approached, I gave Steve Haas an idea for a drawing.

I wanted it to show Dr. Ricky's Nuclear Barbecue, complete with the kind of dark humor that had carried me through the disease. Steve understood my mind well enough to turn the concept into an elaborate piece of art.

The image showed me on the treatment table while Dr. Ricky operated the nuclear barbecue. The details included a spatula and fork, with the phrase, "We have the answer for your cancer."

It was ridiculous, dark, and completely appropriate.

Steve spent many hours creating it. Before I left UCLA, we presented the artwork to Dr. Ricky.

The people around us laughed, and he received it with genuine warmth. Then he asked whether he could have a hug.

After all the moments when I had needed a hand, a hug, or some other reminder that the people treating me saw a human being beneath the mask, the doctor was asking me for one.

I gave it to him, and he gave it back. Doctors are not God, but God placed Dr. Ricky and the rest of the UCLA medical staff in my path, and that path had been paved 40 years before by one of my best friends, Dr. Christopher Wray.

Every time I talk to Dr. Ricky, I say "Thank you for paying attention in school, because I sure as shit didn't."

People say that their doctor is the best. Dr. Ricky is. His staff would always whisper that to me.

The treatment course eventually reached its end. Because I was finishing while hospitalized, there was no public celebration.

There was no crowd of friends waiting in a hallway, no parade, and no dramatic announcement that the battle had been won. I did not stand beside a wall and ring a bell while everyone applauded.

I had seen those moments in videos. Patients rang bells after chemotherapy or radiation, and families recorded the ceremony as proof that they had reached the end.

My ending did not look like that.

The final radiation treatment ended the way the others had. The machine stopped, the technicians returned, and the mask was removed.

Treatment was finished, but nobody could tell me whether the cancer was gone. That answer would not come until the later scan.

Finishing meant only that my body had received everything the doctors could give it for the moment.

The burns remained. The feeding tube remained, and the pain, weakness, sores, low blood counts, and uncertainty remained.

There was no bell because the ending was not an ending.

The hospital prepared to discharge me around the middle of July. I had entered expecting to stay only long enough to control the pain. Instead, I remained through the final stage of treatment.

Leaving required another collection of instructions, medications, supplies, insurance approvals, and equipment. I had to learn how to feed myself through the tube without nurses beside me.

The hospital provided formula that could be pushed slowly into the tube with a large syringe. They also arranged a pump and bag that would deliver nutrition over a longer period, including while I slept at home.

The process was new, and every missing item mattered. The pump required tubing, a stand, formula, and an understanding of how to prevent clogs or deliver the food too quickly.

My friend Kim from Visalia came to take me home. The discharge process became more stressful than either of us expected.

Prescriptions had to be collected, and the insurance company had not yet approved all the feeding-tube formula I would need. The doctors kept working to make sure I would not leave without nutrition.

When the hospital staff loaded my belongings into the car, one necessary piece of equipment was left behind. We did not have the stand needed to hold the feeding bag properly.

I had not wanted to run the feeding pump during the drive home, but Kim insisted I should continue receiving nutrition.

The system did not flow correctly. We pulled over and attempted to call the hospital while trying to understand why the machine was not working.

After weeks in a hospital where nurses handled every tube and alarm, I was suddenly expected to manage the equipment beside a road.

There was no clean transition between being a patient and being responsible for my own care. One moment, medical professionals were checking the equipment. The next, we were driving toward Visalia with a pump that did not seem to be working properly.

Eventually, we reached the house.

The first thing I wanted was to see Sophie, Meg, and Smokey.

They were there, but I had to be careful with them. My immune system was weakened, and even an ordinary scratch could create a risk of infection.

Smokey did not understand why he could not climb all over me in the usual way. Meg and Sophie did not understand the tube extending from my stomach or why my body smelled like a hospital.

They knew I had returned.

I lowered myself carefully and allowed them close without letting their claws catch my skin or the tubing. After weeks of missing them from the hospital, their presence made the house feel real again.

I had imagined that coming home would feel like victory. Instead, I felt like a stranger entering a place that belonged to an earlier version of me.

The house was familiar, but I was not. I had left with a functioning throat and returned thinner, medicated, immunocompromised, and dependent upon a feeding tube.

That first night, I connected the pump and prepared to receive nutrition while I slept. I believed I had assembled everything correctly, although I had no nurse standing nearby to confirm it.

The cats remained close, and I tried to settle into my own bed.

There had been no bell, parade, or final statement that I had beaten cancer. Nobody could tell me whether the treatment had worked, and my body was still carrying the damage it had created.

What I had was the house, the feeding pump beside me, three cats watching every movement, and the knowledge that I had made it home.

For that night, home was enough.

CHAPTER SIXTEEN

The Voice That Stayed

"I ain't changed, but I know I ain't the same."

SONG: ONE HEADLIGHT
BAND: THE WALLFLOWERS

The first morning home should have felt peaceful. I had finished treatment, survived the hospital, and made it back to the house where Sophie, Meg, and Smokey had been waiting for me. There had been no bell or parade, but I was home, and for a few hours, that was enough.

I had spent the first night trying to understand the feeding pump. Formula traveled through tubing into the port in my stomach while I slept. I was no longer surrounded by nurses who could correct a mistake, silence an alarm, or confirm that the machine was operating properly. I had been discharged with bags, syringes, medication, formula, tubing, and instructions that were supposed to turn me into my own medical staff.

I woke up in a familiar room feeling unfamiliar inside my own body. The house looked the way it had before I left, but I had returned thinner, weaker, and dependent upon equipment I had not known existed a few weeks earlier. A tube extended from my abdomen, my mouth and throat were still damaged, and my immune system was weak enough that I had to be careful around the cats I had spent weeks wanting to hold.

They did not understand any of those restrictions. Smokey wanted to climb across me, Meg wanted my attention, and Sophie wanted to settle into whatever routine proved I was staying. I tried to let them close without allowing their claws to catch the feeding tube or break my skin.

I had imagined homecoming as the point when the worst part ended. Instead, it became the point when I realized how much of the medical burden had followed me home.

At approximately 8:30 that morning, the insurance company called.

The person on the line said they knew I had returned home and wanted to ask a few questions. The tone sounded ordinary at first, the kind of polite professional voice designed to make an interrogation appear helpful.

They wanted to know whether the hospital had discharged me or whether I had simply decided to leave. They asked whether I had gone home against medical advice, what medications I had received, and what instructions had been given to me.

I did not know how to answer many of the questions. I had spent weeks being moved between a hospital bed, radiation, chemotherapy, procedures, blood draws, and palliative care. People had placed medications into IV lines and feeding tubes while I drifted in and out of consciousness. I had been sent home with a bag of prescriptions whose names I could not always remember.

I had not designed the discharge plan. I had followed it.

The questions continued. The representative kept telling me to hold on and that everything would be all right, but the reassurance did not match the experience.

I began crying.

I had been home for less than a day. I was alone in the house, connected to a feeding tube, and trying to understand how to care for a body that no longer worked in familiar ways. Instead of receiving one quiet morning, I was being asked to prove that I had left the hospital properly.

"What drugs did they give you?" the person asked.

"I don't know," I said. "I don't know what they fucking gave me."

That was the truth. I had a bag of medication and no interest in being tested on it at 8:30 in the morning.

The conversation lasted approximately forty-five minutes. The longer it continued, the more it felt as though they were searching for a reason not to cover something.

I had entered treatment saying I did not want to spend whatever time I had left fighting insurance companies. I had already been forced into those fights before the first dose of chemotherapy, and now the same system had followed me home.

I wanted one day of grace. One morning without an appointment, an insurance question, a needle, a machine, or somebody asking me to explain what had been done to my body.

They did not give me that morning.

By the end of the call, I was sobbing. The representative continued using the same controlled voice, telling me there were only a few more questions. I wanted to know why none of those questions could have waited until later in the day or been answered by the hospital that had discharged me.

The call ended eventually, but the emotional reaction did not. Even after I placed the phone down, I remained inside the same panic I had experienced during the mask, the darkest nights in the hospital, and now again, the impending doom I woke up with every morning during the pandemic

I was home, but my nervous system had not received the message. The insurance issue was partly connected to the feeding-tube formula. The hospital could justify keeping me admitted because of my medical condition, but obtaining approval for the food I needed at home had become more complicated.

That seemed insane to me. The doctors had placed a tube into my stomach because I could not eat. The purpose of the tube was to deliver nutrition, yet somebody still had to decide whether the nutrition would be covered.

Eventually, large boxes of formula arrived at the house. The cartons were heavy, industrial-looking reminders that food had become medicine.

Before treatment, I chose meals according to taste. I joined the country club largely because I wanted somewhere to eat well when I returned from traveling.

Now calories were numbers written on cartons. Eating no longer involved a plate, fork, smell, or flavor. It involved pouring liquid into a bag or loading it into a large syringe and pushing it slowly through a tube in my abdomen.

I had to learn how quickly the formula could enter without making me sick. I had to flush the tube with water so it did not clog and clean the area where it entered my body. Every connection had to remain secure, especially when I was sleeping.

The process kept me alive, and I hated almost everything about it.

The overnight pump seemed practical. It could provide nutrition while I slept and reduce the number of feedings I had to manage during the day.

After approximately a week, a new problem developed. I would wake in the morning with thick white foam and formula backed up into my mouth. Even though the nutrition had entered directly into my stomach, it was returning through my throat while I slept.

The sensation disgusted and frightened me. My mouth already felt damaged, dry, and unfamiliar. Waking with feeding formula inside it made me feel as though my own body was rejecting the method intended to support it.

I did not want to remain connected to the pump through the night. I did not want to wake with that taste and texture in my mouth, especially when taste itself had become distorted.

I decided I was going to try swallowing again.

The idea was simple, but the act was not. My throat had been burned by radiation, my swallowing muscles had weakened, and my stomach had adjusted to receiving very little at a time. I could not suddenly return to ordinary meals.

I had high-calorie nutritional shakes containing approximately 575 calories each. I poured one into a blender, added yogurt to thicken it, and included a scoop of peanut butter.

The mixture still required effort to swallow. I had to move slowly and remain aware of every part of the process, but I managed to get it down.

That felt like progress.

The doctors wanted me to consume roughly two thousand calories each day. Reaching that target through the shakes could require four or five of them, depending upon what I added.

Before cancer, I could have consumed two thousand calories without thinking about it. After treatment, one shake could feel like a project occupying much of the day.

My stomach had become smaller from weeks without normal food. If I drank too much or too quickly, nausea followed. If I waited too long, weakness and dehydration became worse.

There was no natural hunger guiding me. Taste had disappeared or changed, and appetite had become unreliable. I ate according to what my body required, not according to what it wanted.

The doctors had given me MuGard to coat and soothe the inside of my mouth and throat. It was supposed to make swallowing more tolerable, but it often made me gag or vomit.

Something could be medically designed to help me and still feel impossible to use. That became one of the lessons of treatment and recovery. The fact that a product helped many patients did not guarantee my body would accept it.

The pain medication I brought home felt weak compared with what I had received in the hospital. There, a nurse could administer medication through a line and create relief within seconds. At home, I swallowed pills or liquids and waited, never knowing whether the relief would be enough.

I had wanted to leave the hospital. Once I was home, I missed the certainty that somebody would respond when the pain became unbearable.

The summer heat made recovery more isolating. Temperatures in Visalia rose into the hundreds, and walking outside for long periods was not realistic.

I spent hours inside the house with the curtains closed, the air conditioning running, and the cats nearby. I had once spent so much time traveling that I wished for weeks at home. Now the house sometimes felt like another form of confinement.

The difference between home and the hospital was that nobody entered automatically. There was no nurse checking vital signs, no food tray arriving, and no technician telling me which appointment came next.

I was grateful for the quiet and frightened by it.

My neighbors continued watching over me. Chris & Jenna and their daughters checked in, as did KC & Lauren, Scott & Samantha, Jhenny and Cyrus, and others around the street.

They understood that I had completed treatment but was nowhere near finished with cancer. The body does not immediately repair itself because the radiation machine has stopped.

They brought food even when I could not eat it normally. They watched the cats when I needed appointments or assistance and helped with practical problems that would have felt minor before cancer.

Their support did not arrive as a motivational speech. They were simply present.

That was what I needed most.

Other people frequently told me I was strong or brave. They said God would never give me more than I could handle and assured me that everything would be fine.

I knew those words came from love. I also knew they could make me feel more alone.

Being called strong created pressure to perform strength. Being told I would be fine ignored the fact that nobody had the scan result yet. Telling me that "God gives his strongest soldiers His toughest battles" made me think about the people who had died from cancer.

Had God given them too much?

I did not need anyone to explain cancer, faith, or courage to me. I needed people willing to admit they could not fully understand what was happening inside my body.

The most honest thing someone could say was, "I cannot imagine what you are going through, but I am here."

The second part mattered only if the person meant it.

My neighbors meant it.

The cats did too, although their support came with claws, loud demands, and no understanding of medical boundaries. They followed me from room to room and watched the feeding process as though I had adopted a new and suspicious ritual.

Smokey remained especially close. He had noticed something around my neck before the tumor appeared. He knew what I knew, that I had cancer, and now he seemed determined to monitor every stage of my recovery.

I could not prove that he understood cancer. I knew only that he understood me.

My friend Julie Estrada, whom Donny and I had met a few years before, and who started photographing our shows, would come over every weekend while the teams were out performing, and just hang with me. We would watch hours of Family Guy. Her friendship and dedication to The Killer Dueling Pianos was immeasurable. Although she's not a piano player, she is a patch holder. The center photo on the cover of this book was taken by her.

The chemotherapy had left another problem behind. My fingers and toes became numb, and I developed extreme sensitivity to temperature.

Cold surfaces could feel painful, and heat could become difficult to judge. The same fingers that had spent my life moving across piano keys and guitar strings no longer communicated with my brain in the same way.

The neuropathy frightened me because music required precision. A piano player needs to know where his fingers are without staring at each one. A guitarist needs to feel the pick and understand how tightly he is holding it.

I did not know whether the numbness would improve, remain permanently, or become something I had to adapt around.

I began entering the pool carefully. The doctors had said I could swim with the feeding tube as long as I protected the site and followed the necessary precautions.

The pool had once represented my attempt to provide a life for Red. Later, it became something I reclaimed for myself. Now it represented another test of what my body could tolerate.

The water felt different against skin and nerves changed by chemotherapy. My fingers and toes responded unpredictably to the temperature.

I entered slowly and did not remain for long. Even a brief moment in the water gave me something the hospital had not.

I was back inside my own life.

The feeding tube remained the clearest evidence that I was not free of treatment. It had to be flushed each day, and the skin around it had to remain clean.

I wanted it removed as quickly as possible.

Part of that desire was practical. The tube was uncomfortable, required constant maintenance, and prevented me from forgetting cancer even briefly.

Another part was emotional. H was planning to visit, and I did not want her to see me with a tube extending from my stomach.

The doctors would not remove it simply because I was embarrassed. They wanted evidence that I could maintain enough nutrition by mouth and that removing the tube would not force another procedure later.

They had seen patients rush the process and then lose weight, dehydrate, or require the tube again. Their caution made medical sense.

I still hated it.

H had entered my life again while I was in the hospital. We had known each other in Baltimore more than twenty years earlier, when I was still drinking, taking pills, and behaving in ways that made me incapable of sustaining a healthy relationship.

She had every reason to leave me then. I had not been a good boyfriend, and losing the relationship might have contributed to the chain of events that eventually forced me toward recovery.

During the hospital stay, we began speaking regularly. H told me she had continued thinking about me and wanted to see me.

The conversations gave me something to anticipate beyond medication, tube feeding, and the future PET scan. I began imagining that the relationship might return in a different form now that I had been sober for almost twenty years.

I wanted her to meet the man I had become, but I also wanted her to see the damaged version of me. Red's departure had left me terrified that nobody would remain when life became difficult.

If I ever allowed myself to love someone again, I wanted to know that she could see me at my worst and not immediately run.

Cancer made that desire more intense and less rational.

I began making plans far beyond what the situation justified. My mind had moved from the controlled environment of the hospital into a house filled with uncertainty, medication, loneliness, and the belief that I might still die.

I was not thinking like a healthy man planning a careful future. I was thinking like someone who had recently finished brutal treatment and did not know whether it had worked.

I decided to enclose the back patio and turn it into another room.

The room could serve as an office for H if she eventually moved to California. Until then, it could become my workspace, allowing the kitchen table to return to being part of a home rather than the center of The Killer Dueling Pianos.

The idea itself was not unreasonable. The speed and emotional force behind it was.

I hired people and began the construction before I knew what H and I actually were. I was attempting to build physical space for a relationship that had not yet been re-established.

I had made similar decisions before with the pool and Red. Now I was recovering from cancer, speaking with a woman from my past, and building a room.

The object had changed. The instinct had not.

I also decided to buy an RV.

Part of the reason involved the company. If I returned to performing, an RV could make traveling more comfortable and give me somewhere to rest at outdoor events or during long runs of shows.

I had spent years moving through hotels and trucks without taking real vacations. An RV could create another way to travel and possibly allow me to experience something beyond the work itself.

My friend Rusty, who had sold me my first Harley-Davidson years earlier, was now selling RVs. I contacted him and began the process.

Donny drove me approximately four hours to complete the paperwork and then drove me home again. I was still weak, dealing with neuropathy, managing the feeding tube, and recovering from weeks in the hospital.

He did what he had done throughout cancer. He showed up and drove.

Donny had become more than a partner or employee. He had carried the company while I was hospitalized, brought supplies, cared for my home, checked on the cats, traveled to appointments, and witnessed emotional moments I would have hidden from almost anyone else.

There was no reasonable way to calculate what I owed him.

The RV arrived, and the construction around the house continued. I was creating movement and projects while waiting for my body to heal.

Work had always helped me avoid stillness. Cancer had not removed that habit.

There were practical reasons for what I was doing, but underneath them was fear. If I stopped planning, I had to confront the possibility that there might be no future in which I used the new room or RV.

Making plans was my way of voting for survival.

H came to California near the end of July. I drove to the airport to pick her up even though I still did not feel well.

The heat was intense, the feeding tube remained in place, and my body looked nothing like it had when we were together decades earlier. I was excited to see her and deeply insecure.

More than twenty years had passed since we had stood face-to-face. We were not the same people, although parts of the old connection returned immediately.

She looked beautiful to me. The attraction was still there, and within hours, the physical part of the relationship returned.

It had been years since I had allowed myself that kind of closeness. After Red left, I had protected myself by refusing to become vulnerable with anyone.

For a brief time, H's presence felt like proof that my body had not been completely destroyed. I still carried the feeding tube and treatment damage, but I could feel desire and be desired.

That mattered more than I expected.

The following morning, H said she wanted to leave.

The change was abrupt, and I did not handle it well. I had imagined far more than the visit had promised. In my mind, she had become connected to the new room, the RV, recovery, and a possible future.

To her, the visit did not mean the same thing.

She told me I remained too self-obsessed. Under ordinary circumstances, I might have been capable of hearing part of that criticism and examining it.

These were not ordinary circumstances.

I had spent months thinking about cancer, treatment, pain, insurance, food, medication, survival, and whether my voice would remain. My life had necessarily become focused on my body because nearly every part of my day involved keeping that body alive.

That did not mean I had handled every conversation well or made enough space for what H was experiencing. It meant I was still too emotionally fragile to receive the criticism without hearing it as another complete rejection.

She left.

We spoke after she returned home, but the conversation became an argument. I told her I had been fighting cancer and was not completely myself.

The argument escalated, and I called her a piece of shit before hanging up.

That was not how I wanted to respond. Recovery had taught me better ways to handle anger, and I had been sober long enough to understand that pain did not give me permission to say anything I wanted.

Knowing that did not prevent the words from leaving my mouth.

H later made it clear that she had viewed the visit primarily as a physical encounter, not the beginning of the future I had imagined.

The truth hurt, but it also exposed how much of the story I had written without her agreement. I had converted phone calls and attraction into plans for a shared life.

We were two people with history and chemistry who were not standing on the same emotional page.

I had wanted H to prove that someone could see me at my worst and remain. That was too much weight to place on a brief visit from a person I had not seen in more than twenty years.

Her departure reopened the old wound created by Red. The circumstances were different, but my mind recognized the feeling immediately.

Someone had entered my home, allowed me to imagine connection, and then left.

This time, however, the heartbreak did not exist inside the same emptiness as 2020. The business had not disappeared, the world was not shut down, and I was not completely isolated.

My neighbors remained nearby. Donny remained in my life, the company continued operating, and the cats still followed me through the house.

I had also survived something that had changed the scale of emotional pain. H's departure hurt, but it did not burn like radiation. It did not prevent me from swallowing or require a morphine pump.

That did not make the loss unimportant. It reminded me that pain could exist without becoming the only thing in my life.

I continued trying to eat.

The radiation and chemo had destroyed my taste buds.

Taste returned in confusing fragments. One moment I believed I could detect sweetness, salt, or some familiar part of a meal. The next moment, everything tasted wrong or like nothing at all.

My mind often supplied the memory of flavor before my mouth confirmed it. I could look at food I had loved and almost remember the experience strongly enough to believe I was tasting it.

Then I swallowed and discovered the taste was not there.

Food had become an argument between memory and biology.

I kept experimenting because eating by mouth was one of the paths away from the feeding tube. Some textures worked better than others, and certain flavors were more detectable.

Nothing was consistent enough to celebrate confidently.

The body healed on its own schedule. I could not make taste buds return through effort, money, discipline, or prayer.

That was difficult for someone accustomed to solving problems through action.

I could complete swallowing exercises and consume the required calories. I could hydrate, attend appointments, and follow instructions.

I could not order my nerves, salivary glands, and taste buds to recover by a particular date.

It became a game of not what tastes good, but what doesn't taste like shit.

The waiting became its own stage of cancer.

Treatment was over, but the doctors would not immediately scan me and declare whether it had worked. The tissue needed time to heal because inflammation from radiation could interfere with the results.

The plan was to wait approximately ninety days and then perform a PET scan.

Ninety days is not a long period when viewed on a calendar. It is much longer when the question at the end is whether cancer remains inside your body.

Everyone wanted to speak as though the treatment had succeeded. The odds were favorable, the doctors were optimistic, and the cancer had been attacked with everything they believed would work.

None of that was the same as a scan confirming the outcome.

I had already lived through favorable assumptions being wrong. People had believed the mass in my neck was probably a cyst or something harmless. The doctor had not appeared particularly worried after surgery.

Then the pathology report said cancer...something I already knew months before any tests or surgery. Something I knew during the pandemic was going to happen to me.

Statistics and optimism no longer gave me the comfort they gave other people.

I could hope without pretending to know.

The uncertainty affected every plan. The house addition continued, the RV sat ready, and clients booked future performances. Each of those things assumed I would be alive and capable of using them.

I made the plans anyway.

Recovery had taught me to live one day at a time, but it had never required me to stop placing dates on a calendar. One day at a time meant I did not have to experience the entire ninety-day wait in one moment.

It meant I could live just that day, feed myself that day, care for the tube that day, and make the next responsible decision.

The future could wait for its own day.

The company continued providing evidence that my life had a future. Shows happened without me, and the performers maintained the standard we had built together.

I still answered calls and handled business when I had the energy, but the people around me carried more of the responsibility. Cancer had forced me to learn what I should have understood years earlier: a company that depended entirely on my strength was not a strong company.

The patch had become real in the hospital, and it remained real during recovery.

Donny, Johnny, Steve, Jami, John, and the others did not need me standing over them. They needed clear information, trust, and the freedom to do what they had already proved they could do.

Releasing control remained uncomfortable. It also allowed me to heal without watching the business collapse.

My physical strength returned slowly. There was no morning when I woke and suddenly felt like the person who had performed in Kingsburg before treatment.

Some days I could do more. On others, fatigue arrived without warning and forced me to sit down.

The neuropathy remained in my fingers and toes. My stomach continued reacting to the nutritional changes, and my mouth and throat were still uncomfortable.

I did not feel heroic. I felt damaged and impatient.

People saw me at home, heard me speak, or watched a short video and assumed the worst had passed. They did not see the feeding-tube maintenance, the fear surrounding every new sensation, or the emotional reaction created by opening another insurance envelope.

Recovery from treatment was less visible than treatment itself. There was no machine or hospital bed proving that something serious was happening.

I was simply a thinner man sitting inside his house, trying to learn how to eat.

Knowing what I know, I had all the signs of PTSD.

Music remained nearby.

The guitars were still in the house, and the piano waited where it always had. I had spent the months before treatment asking doctors whether the radiation would take my voice.

Dr. Ricky had shown me the treatment area and the location of my vocal cords. To me, everything in the throat looked impossibly close together.

To him, the distance was enormous.

"I know that seems really close to you," he had said. "But for me, that's a mile away."

I had wanted to believe him, but belief did not protect a voice. Precision did.

The radiation burned tissue near the instrument I had used my entire life, yet the vocal cords were not destroyed.

My speaking voice remained rough, but it remained recognizably mine. It had never deteriorated to the degree I feared.

I began sitting at the piano and testing it.

At first, the act was not a performance. There was no audience, stage, or expectation that I needed to complete an entire song.

I pressed the keys and listened.

The neuropathy made my hands feel different. My fingers did not always communicate cleanly with the instrument, but they could still find the notes.

Then I sang.

The sound was not perfect. My throat had been radiated, my mouth remained dry, and my body was weak. I did not expect the same strength or endurance I had carried before treatment.

What mattered was that the sound came out.

I could hear myself and recognize the person inside it.

For most of my life, I had used music to prove something. As a child, it proved I might belong. In Hollywood, it proved I deserved attention. In bars, it proved I could control a room. Building the company allowed music to become responsibility and service.

After cancer, the first purpose was simpler.

The voice proved I was still there.

I did not know when I would be able to carry a full show. I did not know when the feeding tube would be removed, when taste would return properly, or what the later PET scan would reveal.

Those answers had not arrived yet.

Music did not provide them. It did not certify that the cancer was gone or reverse what treatment had done to my body.

It gave me one thing the disease had failed to take.

I sat in my house with the cats nearby, placed my tingling fingers on the piano, and continued singing. The voice was rough, tired, and recovering, but it was mine. Against everything I had feared, the voice stayed.

EPILOGUE

This Has to Become Useful

"We plow the fields and scatter the good seed on the land.
But it is fed and watered by God's almighty hand"

SONG: ALL GOOD GIFTS
From the Musical Godspell – Stephen Schwartz

At 3:30 on the afternoon of March 28, 2025, a pathology report entered my inbox and divided my life into before and after.

The first line said, "Squamous cell carcinoma positive for p16." There was no doctor beside me, no nurse holding my hand, and no human voice preparing me for what the words meant. There was only an email, an attachment, and the sudden understanding that cancer had entered my life.

I began this story with that moment because it represents more than the way I received my diagnosis. It represents how quickly a human being can become a medical case, an identification number, a pathology result, an insurance liability, or the next name on someone's schedule.

Before opening that report, I was still Ryan. I was a son, brother, friend, musician, business owner, sponsor, neighbor, and the man responsible for Sophie, Meg, and Smokey. I was still answering calls about shows, worrying about payroll, and planning the future of The Killer Dueling Pianos.

The email did not erase any of those identities, but it placed one new word in front of all of them.

Patient.

The medical system needed that word because it had a job to do. The doctors needed to identify the disease, create a plan, and begin attacking it before it spread further. I will remain grateful for the people at UCLA who moved quickly, treated me with kindness, and understood that I was more than the cancer growing inside my neck.

Still, nobody should receive life-changing news without a human being available to explain it.

A person should not spend an entire weekend reading unfamiliar medical terms, searching for answers, and wondering whether death has already entered the room. A cancer diagnosis should not be delivered with the same emotional care as an online receipt.

That is one reason this book exists.

Another reason is the corn-kernel feeling I tried to explain months before the diagnosis. Something near my tonsil did not feel right, but the symptom was easy to dismiss. I was told it might be COVID and then strep throat. Medication was prescribed, and the sensation remained.

I continued working because that was what I had always done. Musicians perform through pain, exhaustion, illness, injuries, and whatever personal disaster happens to be unfolding behind the stage.

The audience has already arrived. The contract has been signed, and the show has to go on.

That attitude helped me build a career. It also made it easier to ignore my body, but I did not.

There are people reading this who have their own version of the corn kernel. It may be a lump, strange sensation, persistent cough, unexplained pain, or something else that feels too minor to justify becoming difficult.

They may have already been told that it is nothing. They may be afraid of looking dramatic, wasting a doctor's time, or hearing an answer they do not want.

I understand all of that. I have spent most of my life believing my needs inconvenienced other people.

Cancer taught me that remaining quiet does not make the problem disappear. It only makes you quieter while the problem continues.

You know your own body better than anyone else. That does not mean every fear is a diagnosis or every symptom is cancer. It means you have the right to continue asking questions when the explanation does not match what you are experiencing.

You are not being difficult by asking someone to look again. You are not wasting time by seeking another opinion. You do not owe anyone an apology for protecting your own life.

I had to learn that lesson repeatedly. I had to demand the CT scan order that had never been sent, ask for help with the MRI anxiety, tell the radiation team when the molded pillow was uncomfortable, and admit that the medication was not controlling the pain.

Every one of those moments activated the same old fear. I thought somebody would be angry with me, and I worried that I would be viewed as demanding or weak.

Most of the time, the people caring for me responded with kindness. They adjusted the pillow, slowed down the mask process, changed the medication, or found another way forward.

When someone did not respond with kindness, I still had the right to speak.

The medical professionals possessed knowledge and skills I did not have. That made them essential to my care, but it did not make me irrelevant to it.

I was the person inside the body.

Cancer also taught me how incomplete the word support can be. Before treatment, I would have said I understood support. I had spent years participating in fundraisers and helping other people's families through difficult situations.

I knew how to arrive at an event, donate a performance, encourage a crowd, raise money, and tell someone I was thinking about them. Those things matter, and I remain proud of every cancer fundraiser The Killer Dueling Pianos has performed.

Then I became the patient.

I learned that support is not one large gesture. It is hundreds of small decisions made by people who could have chosen to remain comfortable somewhere else.

Support was Donny driving me to UCLA, sleeping in the second bed at the Tiverton, carrying the company, and continuing to perform when I could not. It was his hand near me before treatment and his shoulder beneath my face when I came out of the radiation room crying.

Support was Chris recognizing my name on an operating-room schedule and appearing beside me when I least expected it. It was his medical knowledge, friendship, and willingness to guide me through a system I did not understand.

Support was Kevin taking my hand before the first radiation treatment because he understood what I needed without requiring me to explain it through a bite guard and a mask.

Support was the technicians slowing down after witnessing my panic. It was their willingness to cut eyeholes into the mask, play The Beatles, and give me the hugs I was not sure I was allowed to request.

Support was Alex brushing knots out of my hair and helping me take a shower when I could no longer perform ordinary acts independently. It was Kelley traveling across the country, caring for the cats, and remaining near me even when pain made me nearly impossible to live with.

Support was my brother Rick entering the hospital room with a teddy bear. It was my parents encouraging me to use whatever medication was medically necessary without treating it as a betrayal of nearly twenty years of sobriety.

Support was my brothers answering late calls when I said I did not know whether I wanted to continue treatment. It was my sponsor listening rather than trying to perform wisdom.

Support was Kim bringing food, Roger and Celeste opening their home, and friends from different parts of my life returning when they heard what was happening.

Support was Chris and Jenna, their daughters, Casey and Lauren, Scott and Samantha, Jhenny and Cyrus, and the other people on my street becoming the family close enough to walk across the yard. They fed the cats, watched the house, brought food, prayed with me, and continued checking in after treatment ended, and everyone else might have assumed I was fine.

Support was Sophie, Meg, and Smokey remaining beside me without understanding anything about cancer. They did not know why I had disappeared, why a tube extended from my stomach, or why I could not allow them to scratch me.

They only knew that I had returned.

I had more support than many people could imagine, and there were still moments when I could not continue. I had friends, family, financial security, excellent medical care, a successful company, and people willing to cross the country to sit beside me.

I still reached a point where I wanted the pain to stop more than I wanted to live.

That fact stays with me because there are people going through cancer with none of the advantages surrounding me. Some are worried about rent while sitting in chemotherapy. Some have children depending on them and no idea how to explain why a parent is sick.

Some do not have reliable transportation to treatment. Some do not understand the medical language being spoken around them, and others are too frightened to admit that they do not understand it.

Some patients return to an empty home after chemotherapy. Nobody is waiting to bring them food, check their medication, help them shower, or listen when fear arrives in the middle of the night.

A social worker may be the only person who calls them. A nurse may be the only person who touches their hand.

Nobody should have to do this alone unless being alone is what that person chooses.

During treatment, I began imagining an organization called Call Ryan. I do not yet know exactly what structure it would require or how much work and money would be needed to make it real.

The idea is simple. A person facing cancer alone should be able to connect with a survivor, volunteer, or family member who understands the value of being present.

That presence might involve a phone call before the first treatment. It might mean driving someone to chemotherapy, waiting during radiation, helping with groceries, or accompanying a person to cut his or her hair before treatment causes it to fall out.

It might mean sitting quietly without trying to say anything inspirational.

The person would not need to pretend to understand every part of the disease. He or she would need to show up, listen, and remain willing to help.

I learned that many of the things people say to cancer patients are designed to comfort the speaker as much as the patient. People want to believe everything will be fine because the alternative frightens them.

They tell you that you are strong and brave. They say God never gives anyone more than that person can handle and promise that a positive attitude will carry you through.

I know those statements usually come from love. I also know how much pressure they can create.

There were days when I did not feel brave. I felt angry, terrified, ashamed, exhausted, and ready to stop.

When someone called me strong, I sometimes felt responsible for continuing to act strong. It became another performance, except this time the stage was a hospital bed, and the audience was everyone who needed to believe I was winning.

Cancer does not require a patient to inspire anyone.

A patient has the right to cry, curse, question God, hate treatment, feel ungrateful, and admit that the pain is too much. None of those responses represent a failure of character.

The most helpful words may be the simplest ones.

"I cannot imagine what you are going through, but I am here."

That sentence leaves room for the patient's experience instead of replacing it with a slogan. The final three words matter only when the person saying them is prepared to act.

Being there might not be convenient. It may require rearranging plans, listening to the same fear repeatedly, or remaining close to someone who is no longer behaving like the person you once knew.

Pain changes people. Medication changes people, and fear can make a loving person angry, selfish, unreasonable, or emotionally unreachable.

I experienced all of those changes. I was not always gracious to those helping me, and some people witnessed parts of me I wish I had handled differently.

Their willingness to remain did not excuse my behavior. It gave me the chance to survive long enough to examine it.

That is part of what recovery has always meant to me. Sobriety did not transform me into a finished human being. It gave me enough clarity to recognize my behavior and enough time to do something about it.

For nearly twenty years, staying alive meant remaining away from alcohol, pills, cocaine, and the substances that had consumed my life. Then cancer placed narcotics, anxiety medication, and medical cannabis back into the conversation.

I had to reconsider what sobriety actually meant.

The younger version of me used substances to escape life. During cancer, I used medically necessary substances to remain inside it.

The distinction was not always emotionally easy, but it was real. I spoke with my sponsor, parents, and people who had spent decades in recovery. Nobody told me I had failed or lost my sobriety.

They told me to save my life.

Recovery was never supposed to become another method of punishment. It was supposed to offer freedom from the behavior that was killing me.

When cancer became the thing capable of killing me, the purpose remained the same.

Do what is necessary to live.

That did not mean every medication felt safe or comfortable. My body remembered the relief narcotics provided, and part of my mind recognized the rush when the hospital placed the morphine button in my hand.

I had to remain honest about that too.

Honesty has done more to protect my sobriety than pretending temptation no longer exists. I am not immune to addiction because I have remained sober for years.

I am alive because I know I am not immune.

The same honesty belongs in this book. I have not written a clean story about overcoming addiction, building a successful company, defeating cancer, and walking into the sunset as a transformed man.

That is not what happened.

Sobriety did not permanently eliminate insecurity, emotional immaturity, resentment, or my need for control. Financial success did not heal the heartbreak that remained after Red left.

Cancer did not erase those problems by giving me something more serious to think about. Some of them followed me into the hospital, entered the radiation room, and were waiting inside the house when I returned.

Survival is not the same as completion.

I continue to carry damage from everything that happened. My relationship with food changed, my taste became unreliable, and swallowing required effort that once happened automatically.

The chemotherapy left numbness and sensitivity in my hands and feet. My body became tired in ways I could not always predict, and medical calls or insurance letters could return me emotionally to the first morning after the hospital.

I remained uncertain about what the later scan would reveal. Treatment had ended, but the answer had not arrived simply because the final radiation session was complete.

There was no bell because there was no clean conclusion.

I learned to live inside that uncertainty by returning to what recovery had taught me years earlier. I did not need to experience the next ninety days at once.

I needed to live the day in front of me.

On some days, that meant drinking enough calories to move closer to freedom from the feeding tube. On others, it meant flushing the tube, answering a client, sitting beside the pool, or allowing my neighbors to help me.

Sometimes it meant crying without trying to turn the tears into a spiritual lesson.

One day at a time is often presented as a slogan. For me, it became the only practical way to live.

I could not control the future scan. I could not force taste, saliva, nerves, strength, or swallowing to return according to my preferred schedule.

I could complete the exercises, attend the appointments, follow medical advice, and remain honest about what I felt.

The result belonged to another day.

Music was one of the things I could return to without waiting for a scan.

For weeks before treatment, I asked Dr. Ricky whether radiation would take my voice. Donny and I questioned him repeatedly because losing the ability to sing frightened me more than dying.

Dr. Ricky showed me where the radiation would be directed and where my vocal cords were located. To me, everything looked impossibly close.

To him, the distance was enormous.

He told me the radiation could be shaped precisely enough to reach what needed to be destroyed while protecting the instrument I had carried since childhood.

I wanted to believe him, but cancer had taught me not to place complete trust in predictions. I had already been told that the lump in my neck probably was not cancer.

I waited to see what my body would do.

My speaking voice became rough, but it never disappeared. Once I returned home, I began sitting at the piano and testing it.

My hands felt different because of the neuropathy. My throat remained dry, and I did not have the strength or endurance to perform a full show.

I pressed the keys anyway.

Then I sang.

The sound was damaged and tired, but it came out. I could hear enough of myself inside it to know the voice had survived.

I knew if I did not get up and start working out my voice again, set a date to get back on stage, I would never take the stage again.

On September 26th, less than 3 months after leaving the hospital, my body still tingling from neuropathy, light-headed, I took the stage for a fundraiser in Visalia, California and sang the whole 3 hour show.

On November 12th, Donny and I flew to Texas, got into the truck with Tim Georgeff, and performed 3 shows in a row in Richmond, Midland, and Abilene.

I have been touring full time with Donny again ever since that weekend.

For most of my life, music had been connected to my need to prove something. As a child, it helped me feel less insecure. As a teenager, it gave me an identity, and in Hollywood, it fed the dream that attention might finally make me whole.

Later, music became employment, addiction, responsibility, leadership, business, and service. It helped create The Killer Dueling Pianos and provided work for people I loved.

Cancer reduced the meaning to something more basic.

The voice proved I was still here.

It was not proof that the cancer was gone, and it did not mean my body had returned to normal. It was one surviving part of me speaking through everything the treatment had changed.

That voice now has another job.

Ryan's Rockstars began in 2021 as the name of a fundraising team. I entered the campaign believing I lacked the large local family or corporate support available to other candidates.

Then people stepped forward.

Clients opened their homes, friends organized fundraisers, caterers donated food, the Lions Club became involved, and people from the Central Valley treated me like family. My parents donated, Dennis raised money in Ohio, and Donny became the campaign manager.

We raised approximately fifty-seven thousand dollars through private donations. Fifty thousand dollars supported acute myeloid leukemia research in memory of Jennifer Stahl-Doyle.

I did not win the title connected to the campaign. I received the Big Heart Award, but the title was never the most important outcome.

Jenn's name became connected to research that might help another person survive the illness that took her.

Halfway through the campaign, I told Donny we were not finished with Ryan's Rockstars. I did not yet know what the name would become, but it felt larger than one six-week campaign.

Cancer gave that feeling a clearer direction.

I want Ryan's Rockstars to create joyful experiences for children fighting cancer. Children should not have to understand why treatment hurts before they are allowed to experience something that makes them happy.

The experience might be a trip, a party, a concert, a princess arriving at the door, or anything else capable of making that child smile. I do not care whether the idea looks impressive to adults.

The point is the child.

Treatment can make a person's world very small. Days become organized around medication, pain, scans, needles, and medical language.

Joy does not cure cancer, but it can remind someone that cancer has not become the only part of life.

Music has given me more joyful experiences than I can count. It allowed me to travel, meet extraordinary people, build a company, and help raise money for causes larger than myself.

Ryan's Rockstars can become one way of sending that joy somewhere it is needed.

I do not know how quickly the organization can be built or exactly what legal and operational structure it will require. I know only that I have performed dozens of cancer fundraisers over the years and have seen what a room full of people can accomplish when music gives them a reason to gather.

I know the company has a network of performers, clients, venues, and people who have repeatedly shown that they are willing to help. The first Ryan's Rockstars campaign succeeded because ordinary people gave what they could.

That same principle can continue.

The purpose is not to place my name above anyone else's. It is to use whatever recognition I have to direct attention toward children who need it.

Cancer gave me what I jokingly called "street cred," although I would gladly surrender that credibility and everything required to earn it.

I now understand the patient's side of the fundraiser. I understand the mask, the mouth sores, the fear of the scan, the hospital nights, the feeding tube, and the emotional crash that can occur after everyone congratulates you for finishing treatment.

I understand that a patient may not feel grateful, brave, or inspired. I understand that surviving the day might require every bit of energy available.

That understanding creates responsibility.

Service has repeatedly saved my life. It saved me in recovery when helping another person interrupted the endless cycle of thinking about myself.

It helped me after Red left, when I asked God to place someone in front of me who needed what had been given to me. It brought me back toward life through the Ryan's Rockstars campaign when my heart remained black.

Service could not eliminate heartbreak, but it made the pain useful.

I do not believe suffering is automatically noble or necessary. I would never tell another patient that cancer happened for a reason.

There are children in treatment who did nothing to deserve what is happening to them. There are families who lose people despite faith, love, excellent doctors, and every available treatment.

Saying everything happens for a reason can become another way of avoiding the unfairness of what happened.

I did not need cancer to become a better person. There were easier ways I could have learned most of these lessons.

Cancer happened. What I do with the experience belongs to me.

I can allow it to remain only as pain, fear, and damage. Those things are real and deserve to be acknowledged.

I can also take what I learned and place it in service of somebody else.

That is different from claiming cancer was a gift. It was not.

The people who appeared around me were the gift. The hands, phone calls, meals, rides, prayers, medical knowledge, humor, music, neighbors, family, and cats were the gifts.

Cancer revealed their value because it stripped away my illusion that I could handle everything alone.

For years, I believed self-respect came from managing my own problems, making money, leading a company, and remaining useful to everyone around me. Depending on others felt like weakness.

Treatment destroyed that belief.

I could not drive myself to every appointment, operate the business alone, place the feeding tube, administer every medication, or remain calm under the mask without human contact.

I needed people.

Needing them did not make me less valuable. It made me human.

The patch I created for The Killer Dueling Pianos was intended to represent trust, brotherhood and sisterhood. I wanted the people wearing it to understand that commitment meant more than accepting the best available gig.

Cancer tested whether that idea was real.

The patched members carried the company when I could not perform. They protected the clients, covered the dates, checked on me, and continued moving the business forward while I was being fed through a tube in a hospital bed.

The patch did not save my life medically. The people wearing it helped make the life waiting after treatment possible.

The same is true of my family. My parents and brothers could not always be physically present, but I never doubted that I remained part of them.

Rick entered the hospital room carrying a teddy bear, and the sight of my brother released emotions I had been containing for years. He had given me my first drumsticks when I was seven, and now he was beside the bed where I was trying to preserve the life those drumsticks helped create.

Mark, Sean, my sisters-in-law, nieces, nephews, cousins, and longtime friends remained connected to me in whatever ways distance allowed. My family story is larger than the amount of space they occupy in these chapters.

Love is not measured only by the number of hospital visits. Sometimes it is measured by the person who continues answering after the patient calls with the same fear again.

The medical staff also became part of the story. Dr. Ricky protected my voice, but he and the UCLA team gave me more than precise treatment.

They listened.

When I described the MRI trauma, he did not dismiss it. When the mask became overwhelming, the technicians adjusted the process rather than treating me as a failed patient.

The palliative-care team allowed me to speak honestly about pain, death, anxiety, and the desire to be unconscious without immediately reducing those thoughts to a problem that needed to be silenced.

The night nurses entered when I woke screaming and told me they had me. During those moments, I believed them.

That kind of care should not depend upon whether someone is fortunate enough to reach a particular hospital. Every patient deserves to feel seen.

My regular doctor, Paul, while fighting his own cancer, got me to the closest qualified ENT he could in the Central Valley before Chris got the ball rolling at UCLA.

Cancer treatment requires machines, chemicals, scans, and scientific precision. It also requires compassion.

The radiation machine attacked the cancer. The hand holding mine helped me remain beneath it.

Both mattered.

That is another reason the story had to be told in detail. Saying I received radiation for seven weeks would have been medically accurate and emotionally incomplete.

It would not explain the mask fastening my shoulders, neck, and head to the table. It would not show the bite guard, postnasal drainage, fear of swallowing, music playing through the speakers, or the moment when everyone left the room.

Saying I received chemotherapy would not explain the fear of losing my hearing, the insurance denial, the neuropathy, or the decision to use medical cannabis after nearly twenty years away from intoxicating substances.

Saying I was hospitalized would not show Alex brushing my hair, Chris appearing before the feeding-tube installation, or the nurses responding when the pain medication wore off at night.

The details are what make another patient feel less alone.

Somebody may one day read about my panic under the mask and understand that his own reaction does not mean he is weak. Another person may recognize that medically necessary pain medication does not automatically erase years of recovery.

A musician may stop ignoring a symptom because the show can continue without him for one night. A family member may learn to sit quietly instead of telling the patient how to feel.

A doctor or technician may be reminded that one slow minute and a hand placed around another hand can change an entire treatment.

That would make the story useful.

I do not know what the final chapter of my medical story will say. The material available for this book ends while healing and testing remain unfinished.

I will not invent a clean outcome because readers deserve the same honesty I demanded from the people caring for me.

I completed treatment. My voice survived, and I began singing again at home while waiting for answers.

Taste, swallowing, pain, neuropathy, fear, and the emotional damage did not disappear at the same time. Recovery did not follow a dramatic movie schedule, and finishing treatment did not mean I knew whether the cancer was gone.

There was no bell because the story was still moving.

That uncertainty may make this epilogue less satisfying to someone expecting certain triumph.

As of now, my current PET scans are clear, but none of my medical staff says "Ryan, you are cancer-free!" so I don't say "cancer-free."

I will be tested every 3 months for the next 5 years for any return.

Cancer is not in my past. The experience lives with me every day.

Real life does not always wait for the ending to become clear before asking us to decide how we will live.

I can wait for certainty before doing something useful, or I can begin with the life and voice available to me now.

I choose now.

The first time music saved me, I was a child searching for somewhere to belong. It gave me an identity when I did not know how to create one myself.

Later, I used it to chase attention, escape insecurity, and feed an ego that could never receive enough. Addiction became tangled with the stage until I could no longer tell where the performance ended, and the destruction began.

Sobriety returned music to me as a responsibility. Building The Killer Dueling Pianos transformed it into an opportunity for other people.

Cancer has given the music another purpose.

The voice that stayed can speak for the patient afraid to ask another question. It can speak for the recovering addict terrified that accepting pain medication means failure.

It can speak for the person sitting alone after treatment, the child who needs one day that does not feel like cancer, and the family member who wants to help but does not know what being present actually requires.

It can also tell the truth about fear, anger, failure, and the moments when survival does not feel inspirational.

I do not need the voice to sound perfect for it to do that work.

I spent much of my life believing value came from applause. Cancer taught me that the most important audience may be one person who needs to hear that he is not the only one falling apart.

That person may never attend a Killer Dueling Pianos show. They may never know the patch, the company, or any of the professional achievements I once believed defined my life.

They may simply open this book after receiving an email that changed everything.

I hope they understand that they have the right to demand a human explanation. I hope they continue asking questions when something inside their body feels wrong.

I hope they accept help before pain makes the decision for them, and I hope someone nearby is willing to hold their hand without promising an outcome nobody can guarantee.

Most of all, I hope they understand that fear does not disqualify them from survival.

I panicked beneath the mask, cried in the radiation room, screamed for medication, questioned God, and said I no longer cared whether I lived. None of those moments stopped me from completing treatment.

Courage was not the absence of those reactions. Sometimes courage was returning to the radiation room after saying I could not do it.

Sometimes it was pressing the morphine button, admitting I needed a feeding tube, or allowing someone to help me shower.

Sometimes it was drinking another shake when food no longer tasted like food.

Survival rarely looked the way I expected. It was not one heroic act. It was thousands of undignified, frightened, ordinary decisions.

Recovery had always worked the same way.

I did not rebuild my life through one grand transformation. I did it by continuing to show up, tell the truth, make amends, keep commitments, and do the next right thing when I understood what that thing was.

Cancer did not change the formula. It changed the circumstances in which I had to practice it.

The next right thing now is to use the voice that remained.

It is to build Ryan's Rockstars into something capable of giving children and families moments of joy. It is to continue exploring Call Ryan so that fewer patients face treatment without companionship.

It is to use music, business, recovery, and the community surrounding me for more than personal success.

It is to keep telling the truth even when the truth does not make me look strong.

This book is part of that work.

I cannot make the diagnosis email more humane by rewriting what happened to me. I cannot remove the mask, restore the months of pain, or give Jennifer the years she should have received.

I cannot change the people who left or undo the nights when I asked God not to let me wake up.

I can decide what happens to those experiences after they pass through me.

They can remain wounds I protect from the world, or they can become a doorway through which someone else finds help.

For most of my life, I believed purpose was something I would discover after achieving enough. I searched for it in Hollywood, bands, money, leadership, relationships, business growth, and applause.

Purpose was not waiting at the end of success. It was present each time I used what had happened to me to help another person.

That may be the most honest understanding of my life I have reached.

The addiction has to become useful. The failures have to become learning experiences, and the heartbreak, sobriety, company, patch, cancer, voice, and every hand that held mine have to become useful.

Otherwise, they remain only things that happened.

At 3:30 on March 28, 2025, an email told me I had cancer. It did not tell me what the experience would mean.

That part was left for me to decide.

My voice is still here, and it has work to do.

This has to become useful.

Photographs

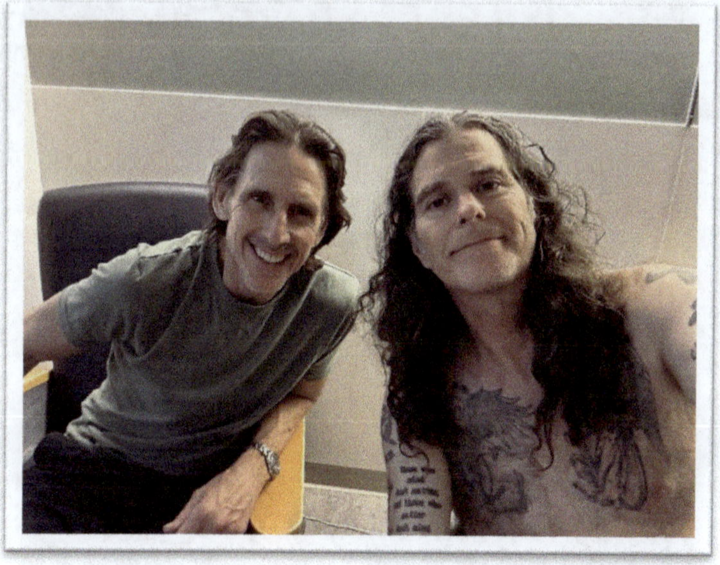

Dr. Chris Wray and Ryan Bueter at UCLA Hospital 6/28/2025

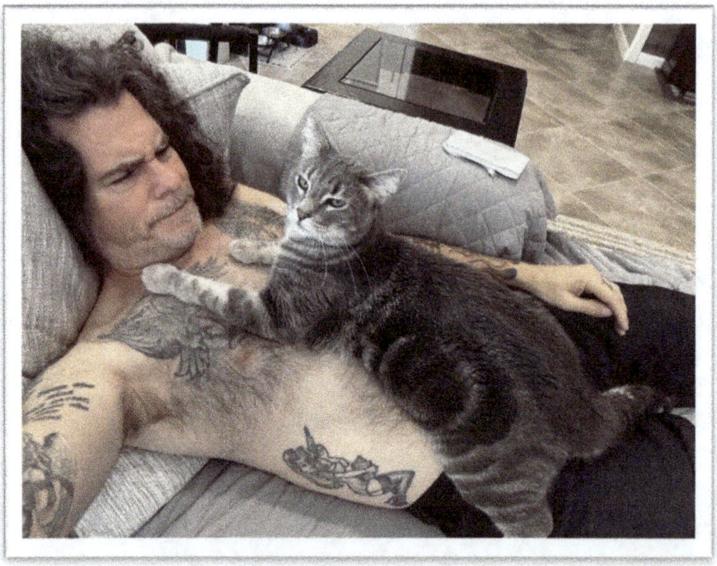

Ryan Bueter and Smokey

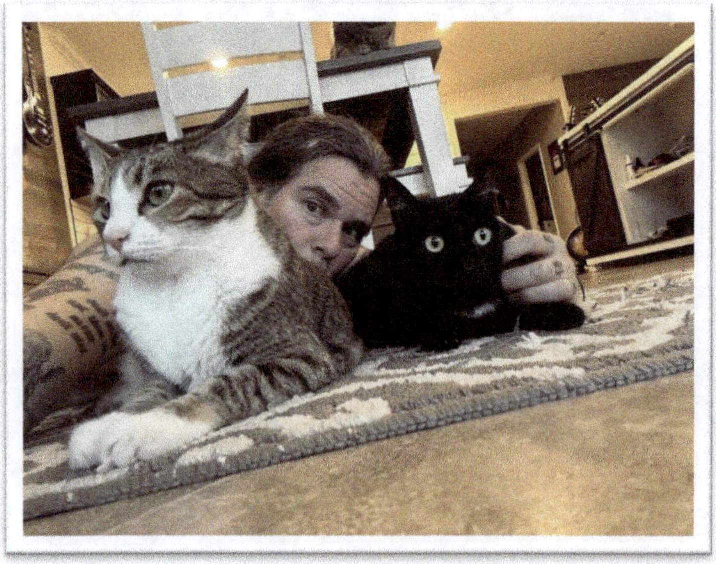

Meg, Ryan, Sophie.

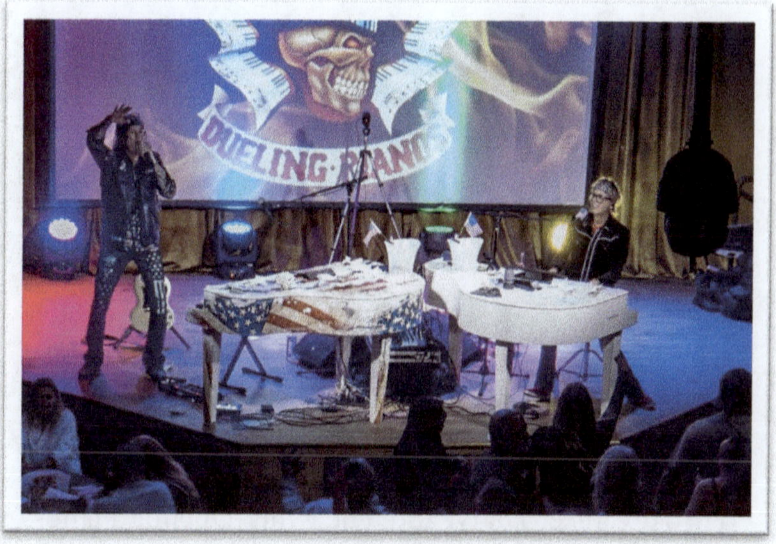

The Killer Dueling Pianos: Ryan Bueter & Donny Scott

Follow Ryan Bueter, Throat Cancer Diary, and The Killer Dueling Pianos

Ryan Bueter

Instagram: @RyanBueter

Facebook: facebook.com/RyanBueter

Throat Cancer Diary

Website: www.throatcancerdiary.com

The Killer Dueling Pianos

www.DuelingPianosForHire

Instagram: @the_killer_dueling_pianos

Facebook: facebook.com/TheKillerDuelingPianos

TikTok: @TheKillerDuelingPianos

Book cover photos: Front-cover center photo and back-cover photos by JME Photography/Julie Estrada.